What's Wrong With Mommy?

Ride The Wave of Postpartum Depression With a Mother of Nine

JoAnne Diaz, MOM
Marriah Publishing

© Copyright 2016

All rights reserved. No part of this book may be reproduced in any form
without prior permission from the publisher.

Marriah Publishing
122 Manners Road
Ringoes, NJ 08551

ISBN # 978-1-945853-02-9

Dedication

First and foremost, I dedicate this book to God and to The Blessed Mother who saved me through both bouts of postpartum depression and who save me every day. For my high school creative writing teacher John Smith who instilled a love of writing within me. For my darling husband, Nicholas, who is taking care of me through this illness. For our beloved children who ride the wave of postpartum depression: Peter, Anthony, Maria, Bella, Nicholas and Thomas, Andrew, Joseph, Philip (and for any other future children!). For my parents, Bel-Mehr and Beaupa who are always there for me no matter what. For my sister, Julie, who saved me by first calling me out on this illness. For my spiritual director, Father Lope, who helped me from afar while I battled this postpartum depression beast. For Colleen Kelly and Jeanne Murphy of Jeanne Murphy PR who helped me fulfill my dream of being an author. For Alexa who gave me her valuable artistic input. For Tina who watched the children so I could write this book. For my BFF, April, who always keeps me grounded and tames the wild horse within me! To Chardonnay, my other BFF, thank you; just thank you! And for everyone who helped us during this time. For all of you who have been asking me for a book, this book is for all of you.

Disclaimer: This book is not intended as a substitute for the medical advice of physicians. The reader should regularly consult a physician in matters relating to his/her health and particularly with respect to any symptoms that may require diagnosis or medical attention.

Introduction

If you are reading this book it is likely due to one or several facts: you're a mom, you have diagnosed (or non-diagnosed) postpartum depression (also referred to as PPD), or you're simply curious about the life of a mom of nine children currently under the ages of nine (or, maybe all of the above!).

My story, I'd say, is a simple one: I was raised in a good Catholic family. I wanted to be a mom all my life until I had a deep conversion. I thought God was calling me to the religious life so I decided to try that out for a little while. It didn't work out but in the end, it was all providential.

A few years after I tried the religious life, I decided to date again. I met my husband through several people from my Church. We had actually seen each other for several years but we were both dating other people. We both agreed to a "blind" date and three weeks later we were engaged and three months later we were married. Fast forward and we have been married ten years and have nine beautiful children. We had all of our children back-to-back and yes, if you have done the math you've got that right: we have a set of twins in there!

I will be honest and say that I had never had postpartum depression until my fourth child. I didn't ever recognize the signs of it. I thought one had to actually be depressed to have an illness that included the word depression. I was dead wrong. Luckily I had someone watching out for me and I survived my first bout of postpartum depression. After that time passed, I wanted to write a book on it but never got to it. Hopefully you won't mind since I was a little busy! People had asked me for years to write a book on how I do it all and so I started but never finished. I am here today writing this book -a new book solely dedicated to postpartum depression- because I just experienced my second bout of postpartum depression after the birth of my ninth child. I knew the book could not wait so here it is. Please "enjoy" it and take it or leave it for what it is worth. I am a mom; that is all. I am not a doctor. I am not a medical professional though I would like to be at one point. This is my story and I am so glad to share it with you in the hopes that it can help you!

Postpartum "Depression"? No, Postpartum Syndrome	1
Researching Postpartum Depression	8
Self-Masochism and The Precursors to My Second Bout of Postpartum Depression	11
The Day postpartum Depression Slapped Me in The Face	16
Progesterone: The Hormone Pill Fallen From Heaven	21
The "Other" Doctor Intervention	24
Work Life Balance: Be Open With Your Boss	27
Help and Support: When Mom Needs A Babysitter	29
How Do You Stop When You Can't?	32
Spiritual Help And The Wild Horse That Can't Be Tamed	34
Don't Take Anything For Granted	38
Baby Steps	41
Face Your Fears	43
Go Off The Grid and Just Say No!	46
Irrational Thinking, Dangerous Objects, and The Goldfish That Had To Go	49
Who's That In The Mirror? Will I Ever Be Normal Again?	54
Do You All.The.Time	59
Never Run Out of Wine. Like EVER. & Self-Medicating	62
Charting Hell	64
What's Your Trigger? Don't Pull it! Listen To Your Body; It Speaks!	69
Oh Crap! Now I'm depressed!	72
Who's talking about Postpartum Depression? No one, that's who	75
Dads Have Postpartum Depression Too	79
Yes, We Would Still Have More and More and More	81
Conclusion	83
Addendum: Poems, Songs, and Blogs That Saved Me	86

CHAPTER 1

Postpartum "Depression"?
No, Postpartum Syndrome.

Let's first start off this chapter with what postpartum baby blues is. According to The Mayo Clinic, these are the symptoms of baby blues:

Signs and symptoms of baby blues — which last only a few days to a week or two after your baby is born — may include:

- Mood swings
- Anxiety
- Sadness
- Irritability
- Feeling overwhelmed
- Crying
- Reduced concentration
- Appetite problems
- Trouble sleeping

Now I personally had (and still have) every symptom on this list except for sadness. I am normally the happiest girl in the world. If I am sad, it is only because I have this illness! So if I still have this at seven weeks postpartum what does that make me? An extended baby blue gal? Let's see...

Now here is what The Mayo Clinic defines postpartum depression as:

Postpartum depression may be mistaken for baby blues at first — but the signs and symptoms are more intense and last longer, eventually interfering with your ability to care for your baby and handle other daily tasks. Symptoms usually develop within the first few weeks after giving birth, but may begin later — up to six months after birth.

Postpartum depression symptoms may include:

- Depressed mood or severe mood swings

- Excessive crying

- Difficulty bonding with your baby

- Withdrawing from family and friends

- Loss of appetite or eating much more than usual

- Inability to sleep (insomnia) or sleeping too much

- Overwhelming fatigue or loss of energy

- Reduced interest and pleasure in activities you used to enjoy

- Intense irritability and anger

- Fear that you're not a good mother
- Feelings of worthlessness, shame, guilt or inadequacy
- Diminished ability to think clearly, concentrate or make decisions
- Severe anxiety and panic attacks
- Thoughts of harming yourself or your baby
- Recurrent thoughts of death or suicide

Untreated, postpartum depression may last for many months or longer.

My first thought after reading this is trust me if you Google to your heart's content, you will see that it actually can last up to a year. If you talk to doctors and moms, they say two years, maybe even longer. For me I never had excessive crying, depression, problems bonding with baby, withdrawing from family and friends (ok well in a normal way! lol), anger, fear that I am not a good mother, feelings of worthlessness, shame or inadequacy. I felt guilty because I felt like I put myself in the situation from doing too much. Other than that, this was DEAD ON for me. YUP.

So now that we know what the baby blues and postpartum depression are, let me tell my story. My sister and I have secretly renamed the term Postpartum Depression to Postpartum Syndrome. We feel this is more accurate (at least in my case!) because the word "depression" is very misleading.

When I hear the word "depressed" I immediately think "sad." But here is what the dictionary states depression as:

- a state of feeling sad

- a serious medical condition in which a person feels very sad, hopeless, and unimportant and often is unable to live in a normal way

- a period of time in which there is little economic activity and many people do not have jobs

In my particular case if I felt sad or hopeless it was only because of the postpartum symptoms! And it was not all the time. It was, after having a great week, having a bad day and wondering where it came from and hoping I had been over the worst part but maybe I wasn't.

But I will never forget the day my sister came to me. I had four children ages four and under. I worked and managed it all just fine, or so I thought. One day my sister, who is a nurse, came and had to have a serious talk with me. She brought her child to watch my children so we could actually talk. That was a red flag because unfortunately we never had time together alone. I remember her sitting me down and telling me she thought I had Postpartum Depression. What were the telltale signs for my sister? The blankness in my look. The detachedness from my kids. I was almost four months postpartum so I didn't think anything of it. I was actually mad at her for being so presumptuous.

However, as it always happens with my sister and me, once she left and after I had gotten the kids to bed I Googled. Oh yes, I Googled and Googled some more. In hindsight I wish I would have listened to the doctors and not Googled. I knew right away from the results that I had postpartum depression. I stood corrected. I realized that my anxiety was not a normal anxiety but a postpartum anxiety. That turned into mind racing and suicidal thoughts as well as thoughts of harming my baby or the children.

The next day I called my sister and gathered with her and some of our mutual friends, some of whom were nurses or in the medical field; all of them were my support team. They are a family to me. They advised me to call my OBGYN so I did right then and there on a Saturday. I couldn't believe the office was even open. I did it; I took the big step, eating humble pie and I said, "I believe I have postpartum depression." If you know me you know I do not like to admit when I am wrong. I think I am right on everything, so the fact that I reached out and asked for help was a huge thing for me. Do you know what my doctor, an older male, said? He said, "No, you are almost four months postpartum. You don't have postpartum depression; it's probably just all those kids running you ragged!" Click. Click? In mind I was saying more than click click click to him for sure! I was floored. So I went back to my support team who were there and told them the news. The medical sector told me to call my other doctor, my family doctor. So I did. Once again I was floored that the office was open on Saturday. Was this a secret they had been keeping all along? Anyway, the moment I explained to the secretary what I thought I had, she booked me right then and there.

I arrived at the doctor's office and I filled out the evaluation for postpartum depression. I talked. I talked a lot. I was sleep deprived. My mind raced. I had irrational thoughts. I had mood swings. I was afraid. But because I was always going going going I never stopped to see it or Google it! I just rolled with it as most moms do. We are wired to work when we are sick, etc. No biggie, right? No, wrong! The doctor said I definitely had it and she suggested a therapist and Zoloft. I am not one to take drugs unless I really believe I need them, like say the epidural (all hail the epi!), so for me to have them call the script in before I had even left the building was huge. However, when I got home and yes, Googled Zoloft I said hell-to-the-no I am not taking that! Side effects: suicidal thoughts, anxiety, etc. Oh yes, that is all I need is for something to intensify my symptoms. No thanks buddy. So I went back to my sister the nurse. And it is a miracle of God for me to share with you that a very simple recipe she cooked up worked for me: super b-complex pills (intravenously if you can get it), vitamins, a lot of water and a healthy diet, exercise, sleep (key!), taking it easy and asking for as much as help as you can (paid help or not!). I did that faithfully and if the laundry piled up it did, if the house was dirty it was ok, but as long as I napped when baby napped and slept as much as possible and did everything else, it worked for me. Within a few months I was back to normal. If the highest level of DEFCON is a five I would say that what I had after this pregnancy was DEFCON two. It was not very severe though it did feel like hell at times. Regarding the therapist, I never went to one only because I have always had a spiritual director, a priest, who helps me with anything that I am struggling with be it mental, physical or spiritual.

CHAPTER 2

Researching Postpartum Depression

I am the type of person who, while I love to read blogs on the internet, when it comes to reading a book I actually like a hard copy. I know, call me old school but it's the truth. So after I discovered I had postpartum depression the first time around and after my sister and I worked on my holistic plan of getting me better the first thing I did is went to the book store. I had Googled a lot and read a lot online but I wanted to read a book that would help me. I was absolutely floored when I arrived at the bookstore and there was virtually nothing there on the bookshelf. I skimmed the titles and just kept thinking no, no, no! And then there it was, the most beautiful title I had ever seen (for that moment in time): Female Brain Gone Insane, with the subtitle An Emergency Guide for Women Who Feel like They Are Falling Apart. Yes! Yes! YES! That was exactly what I was experiencing. I had felt like my brain had gone insane. The nights when I was overtired but could not sleep and I could not shut my mind off; those nights I felt like I was falling apart! I started reading this book (which was written by a nurse) and I felt so much relief. The book talks a lot about hormones and nutritional balance. The emphasis of the book was treating whatever hormonal balance you have naturally and/or with hormone replacement therapy. So yeah, it was the book for me. I highly recommend it.

Sometime later, I do not recall how I stumbled upon it but Brooke Shields wrote a book back in 2005 called Down Came The Rain with the subtitle My Journey Through Postpartum Depression. I personally don't like the title only because for me rain is soothing and it helps things grow, but I did understand why she named it that way. At any rate, I can say without a doubt I never in my life read a book that fast. I read it in two days! I was totally enthralled by it because she mentioned so much of what I was going through. Her book is a personal story and it is raw but if you want something that is non-medical I highly recommend it. After you read it you will know that postpartum depression is real and if you are going through it you may relate to her story, even if not to everything she writes.

With the second bout of postpartum depression I headed back to the bookstore to see if there were any new books that were out. There were a few but none with a title or subtitle that included postpartum depression and that is what I was specifically looking for.

I did purchase a few books that were hormone related and were written by doctors. In the end I returned them because when I got home and read their sections on postpartum depression I was a bit mad (at them). One talked about owning your mood. Ok, I get it but as one dealing with postpartum depression, newsflash: you can't control it! Especially if you want to control it naturally. Sure, you can do things to distract you but the "mood" remains because your hormones are still out of whack.

Another author talked about hugs not drugs. While I do agree that hugs are great and there is a health benefit to them (it is proven) some people need more than hugs! Some people need drugs! I love medical science and I take medications when I need to but I am not one to pop a pill just because the doctor recommends it. I research it, I see if I can manage it holistically and if I can, great! And if I can't I pop the dang pill with no regrets.

Yet another author starts off her postpartum depression talking about it as if it is only depression. She doesn't mention that hey, guess what, some women can have postpartum depression and not be depressed! Like me! Where is the information on the other symptoms like anxiety, mind racing, suicidal thoughts, etc.? It is kind of key if you're going to have a postpartum section in your book. Just sayin'. I will say this about her book though, she discussed things I had not thought about, such as nursing or lack of nursing and how it can cause your hormone levels to shift. That was a great take-away from her book. And like the first book I mentioned, Female Brain Gone Insane, this author talks about testing all of your different hormones to see which one you are lacking in.

As with any book, this book included, you take it or leave it for what it is. Some things may help you and some things may not help you.

CHAPTER 3

Self-Masochism and The Precursors to My Second Bout of Postpartum Depression

Since I experienced postpartum depression with my fourth I knew what to do (or not to do) with the pregnancies, labors, and deliveries of the next four children. With my last pregnancy I was doing ok until we decided to buy a home. We had searched for over three years for the perfect home and we finally found it! The only problem was it was February and the baby was due at the end of March. The other problem was I was going to have to rent out our home. The realtors didn't think I could do it but because I am perfectionist and masochist by trade I got 'er done right away. I posted an ad and the next day I found my renter!

You can imagine that since I try not to do anything half-assed I had to write my own lease. That took forever but I wanted to make it bulletproof and it was. I joked and I said I would never ever sign a lease like that! Did I need to do it? Probably not but I am a psycho.

So after we got the rental part done we moved forward with inspections and all. Everything went swimmingly. At first my realtor suggested closing in the middle of April. I agreed because of course I could have a baby and move a week later. I was super-mom as they call me. I could do it. But then she suggested why not close on April 1st because then I could move slowly over a month's time. That sounded logical and is logical if executed. But masochists, at least this one, aren't logical. We decided to close on April 1st. At the same time of renting the house, packing and fixing the house, etc. we had a major personal situation occur in our family. Most people don't even know about it to this day. That situation landed me in the emergency room at thirty-five weeks pregnant. I was contracting every five minutes for hours. I told them I knew what it was. It was stress induced and I was likely dehydrated. I was dehydrated because after they jacked me up with fluids for hours on end the contractions stopped. I went home to "take it easy." Yeah right. No mother or father of eight kids and a bun in the oven ever takes it easy. Like ever? No, like EVER.

To be honest the personal situation could have cost me my marriage. It could have broken our family up. And no, for inquiring minds, this had nothing to do with him or me cheating on one another. However, our marriage was built on Christ and survives by Christ and so we made it. It was the roughest time in our marriage but we made it and we've actually come out better.

I asked my doctor if I could be induced on March 20th so that I would have some time to "rest" before the baby came. Since I was 39 weeks along it was legally okay to induce me and since I had been induced with all of my children except my twins he agreed to induce me.

Everything went great with the labor and delivery and I was happy as could be. I felt great now that the baby was out. I was so happy because in a few days we would be in the home of our dreams. Life couldn't be better, right? Right until two days later while I was still in the hospital I got the worst call of my life. It was my realtor telling us that there was a problem and she didn't know if we would get the house. Looking back on it now I believe that that is when the postpartum depression started. Why? Because after that I could not sleep, I was worried all the time, I was on the phone or email all the time trying to get the damn house. It wasn't anyone's fault. It was the system but dang it, the system was going to have to rectify it because I became like Scarlet O'Hara from Gone With The Wind. "As God is my witness I will never go hungry again!" I will get that house, the house that I promised my children. I didn't care how many hoops I'd have to jump or how many fiscal ladders I had to climb to get that house but I was going to do it. And literally three days before closing I did it. We did it. Between the realtor, the financial person, and my husband, we did it.

I was still in the hospital when I got the call because the baby had jaundice so we were just waiting for him to be released. While I was in the hospital I saw one of my old doctors (from the practice I left). I was so very happy because I had always loved her and wanted to tell her why I left. So there we stood in the hall and I explained to her what had happened with the other doctor saying I did not have postpartum depression and she shook her head. I told her that honestly I would have left anyone because my new doctor, Dr. Kyle Beiter of The Gianna Center in New Brunswick, New Jersey was a devout Catholic man who also had a big family. He promotes The Creighton Method of Natural Family Planning so I waited a long time to get in as one of his new patients. He also treats women's fertility and health in a natural way and that is another reason why I wanted to go to him. The doctor from my old practice understood and we parted ways joyfully.

But...you know how females are? We can't keep our mouths shut. Secret? What is a secret and is your BFF to be excluded in a secret too? So within an hour I had three nurses in my room doing a postpartum evaluation because they had just talked to my old doctor. Really? Like really? UGH. Keep in mind this was before the call from my realtor's company. I looked at them and said, "Trust me. I know if I have postpartum depression and I don't." I believe that one reason I did not have it there yet was because I was sleeping and resting a lot thanks to the fact that I sent the baby to the nursery at night so I could get a solid stretch of sleep. At any rate this, the reaction of the nurses, just goes to show you how some medical staff take this illness very seriously. I was grateful to them but I was ok, I really was. They should have talked to me the day after I got the house problem!

So now that that house problem was settled (and keeping in mind that I live on masochism) I decided to get the baby baptized and throw a party at my house. The house that was not packed up fully because we had stopped packing thinking we were going to lose it. What the hell was I thinking? Who knows?

The baptism was over so what was next? Besides moving? Well, date night of course...oh and selling stuff on Craigslist...oh and planning my 40th birthday party...oh and planning my son's 1st Holy Communion party...oh and scheduling the new house blessing. Do you see where I am going with this? I was setting myself up for postpartum failure and clearly I didn't care. I wasn't thinking clearly, clearly. Ha!

CHAPTER 4

The Day Postpartum Depression Slapped Me in The Face

We went to the house closing sleep deprived. I felt it. The day before closing we had loaded two hauls with almost all of our home's contents. But I knew, like Dory from Nemo, I had to just keep swimming so I did. After closing we went to finish the rest of the move and if you can believe it or not we actually slept in the new house (with the other house being completely emptied) the night we closed. Our first home was ours for ten years and if you have ever seen the show Hoarders I can tell you that I am an organized hoarder and shopaholic. See a tank top in one color you like; buy them all! Money's no issue/concern/matter (especially when it's on sale at the local thrift store). Want a Thomas engine? I'll buy them all for you because I get them at the consignment sale for one third of the cost! So yeah, there was a lot of stuff!

The second day in the house was a blur. We had people there helping us. We continued to be sleep deprived. Wine is my go-to "drug" so I was also drinking a lot of wine to get through it. As a side note, I just want to clarify that I do not drink and breastfeed. If I have a drink I abstain from breastfeeding until the alcohol is out of my body. The next day was Sunday and I knew that my son had to altar serve. I knew that we both had to go to

Mass because after all it is Sunday, a holy day of obligation and even though I had just had a baby two weeks before that I thought I had to go. I didn't. I was not even thinking.

So I plop my son in the car and take him to church. On the way to the church I called my parents like I do every morning and for whatever reason my mom decided to give me a lecture on several things. I flipped my lid. I hung up on her. That conversation (which was extremely stressful) was the first trigger. It's the one that set me spiraling out of control.

We walked in the door and I got my son to where he needed to be. I looked at my priest who looked at both me and my son like "what's up?" My son said he was just tired. I said I was tired from the move, which he already knew about. Off to serve the Mass they went. And then, it was as if there was too much going on at once for me to handle. The singing, all the people, it was way too much stimulation for me so I walked out into the foyer. I leaned on the wall, kissed the crucifix on my rosary, and begged God for help. And then I literally crumbled to the floor and cried. I was exhausted. I was sleep deprived. I was done. I was rational enough to think it may not look good - me sitting on the floor crying - so I got up and went to my car. I sat there hoping to sleep. I could not. I texted my babysitter and her mom who were in the Church so they knew to send my son out. My sitter walked out and she could tell by looking at me that I was not right. She asked me if I could drive. I said I was not sure. I knew it was four miles to my new home so I sucked it up. My son talked to me on the way home about life and whatnot, and that kept me distracted.

We arrived at the new house and I knew I needed sleep. I went to bed. I could not sleep. My mind was racing. I could not remember if I had eaten. I knew I had coffee only because I had posted it, like everything, on Facebook. But did I eat? No. So I asked my hubby for crackers. He brought them up. I could not eat them. I needed to pump so I pumped. After all, the masochist must keep up her supply for her baby (who she wasn't even really nursing) and so she doesn't get the return of her cycle and get pregnant, right? Right! And then, right then and there it all came crashing down on me. And I knew it. I knew it was postpartum depression.

After I recognized it and yelled at myself because I knew, or thought, my psychotic control freak actions had caused it. I tried to think clearly and couldn't. Something else was wrong, really wrong. Was it my thyroid? OMG, they cut my thyroid pill. Maybe it's that. Maybe I am dying. Maybe it's my blood pressure. OMG what is it?

I called my husband and told him to call the police. I told him I needed to go to the hospital. He knew I was having a panic attack and told me I did not need to call the police. Outside of minor panic or anxiety attacks with my first bout of postpartum depression I had never had attacks. He argued with me and eventually he offered a Xanax. I never take drugs so for me to say yes was huge. I took it and he called the police.

The police took forever. I was thinking I could have been long gone by now. I left in an ambulance and told my husband to get a sitter and meet me at the hospital. He arrived and by then I had already self-diagnosed myself to the nurse: I know what I have. I have severe postpartum depression with a side of sleep deprivation and a side of dehydration. I wanted them to give me a pill to knock me out for days and hook me up to an IV of ever-flowing liquids. They didn't but they did agree with my self-diagnosis, especially after they learned that I had just had my ninth child and learned that my oldest was nine and, oh yeah, that we just moved into a new house. They gave me a script for Xanax since it did help and told me to "rest" and follow up with my OBGYN. I was in and out within thirty minutes, no joke. Thanks, a lot...why am I here?

I arrived at home to a house full of worried people. I explained what happened. I don't remember much of that day but I do remember my friend talking about her postpartum psychosis (Google that one! Wait, DON'T Google it. You don't wanna know.). I was totally freaked out in my head. And then I remember my friend Dennis telling everyone that this was the last thing I needed, all this talking, she needs to go to bed! Amen, brother! So they left and I went to bed.

But again, alas, I could not sleep. I could not shut my mind off. I kept hearing Alleluia in my head over and over and over again like a record player, a broken record player that won't shut off. I began freaking out again. I cried. I called for my husband who was mad that I wasn't asleep. Really? You think you are mad that I am not sleeping? How the hell do you think I feel? It's like being in a desert dying of thirst. You see the water and you know you need it but you can't reach it! He gave me another Xanax and I called my OBGYN.

My OBGYN was at the hospital but he called me right back. I explained what happened. He questioned my thoughts. I admitted that I have had suicidal thoughts. I have thought about hurting my children BUT I told the doctor that I know and recognize that they are irrational and so I do not act on them. My doctor uttered one word, one word that I had totally forgotten about. When I heard that word it was like a breath of fresh air. The word was Progesterone.

CHAPTER 5

Progesterone: The Hormone Pill Fallen From Heaven

When my twins were five months old or so I had a girlfriend who was helping me at my house. She would come to babysit or clean. We would chat because she worked for The Gianna Center in Pennsylvania. She was a receptionist there but helped patients a lot in general and was also teaching Creighton classes. She had warned me if ever I had more children and had postpartum depression to ask my doctor about progesterone shots or capsules. She said she has seen it help a lot of women suffering with postpartum depression. She even said she would take it even if she weren't struggling with it!

Unfortunately for me I had totally forgotten what she said. I had my eighth baby and all was fine. But who knows, maybe if I would have taken it would have helped me feel better overall. At any rate, when my doctor uttered those words I immediately said YES. I got off the phone with him and waited for my husband to go CVS. He ran out later that evening after he put the kids to bed and it was closed. CLOSED? But my old CVS was open 24/7. Yeah, well not this one. I had to wait overnight? OMG I thought I was going to die. I actually took another Xanax because the anxiety was too much for me.

The next day my husband was due to go back to work. I was due to go back to work. Yes, if you have kept up (I can't keep up with myself like ever) I was three weeks postpartum and two days in my new house; the house that was so trashed we couldn't find underwear for the kids for weeks so we put Pull-Ups on them. But I was a contractor and I am paid hourly and I do not get paid time off so yeah, I had to go back. Well needless to say I couldn't so I postponed it, only checking in every so often. My husband took the day off. He went to get my progesterone. I took it and to be honest it was not immediate. It took many hours to kick in and I felt better. I was not perfect but I felt better. Before the progesterone I was like running on 10% but with the progesterone I felt like a solid 30%, which is actually good for me being a mom who never stops.

There are side effects with taking progesterone. I took the capsules and I can tell you it made me feel dizzy. My prescription was for two pills in the morning and two at night but my doctor did tell me that I did not have to take two each time; if I wanted to take one in the morning and one at night that was fine. Long-term progesterone does not seem to have many side effects.

For me I eventually ended up weaning myself to two pills a day and then, without any intention whatsoever I went to one a day when I went to nap and then I completely stopped. I was on progesterone for a total of less than four months. For me personally I stopped when I felt normal again and I could tell by my charting that my body was returning to its normal cycle. I can't explain it but I just felt it. And it ended up being amazing because I was right! As my body went without the progesterone capsules it was back to making it normally (and the amount I needed) all on its own!

I am now a full-blown promoter of progesterone and if we have more children I will be sure to go on progesterone right after birth until I feel normal again. I believe this saved my life! I know it has saved others. Maybe it can save you or someone you know who is also experiencing postpartum depression?!

CHAPTER 6

The "Other" Doctor Intervention

During this time around it took me so very long to feel normal. To be honest I am still not there but that is ok because I know I will be. I had many people come to me and tell me to go to my doctor, my normal doctor, and get tested for a regular full workup. I do this every year on my own. When I have a baby I usually do the full blood work after 6 weeks postpartum but in my case I felt that I needed to do it sooner.

So I went to my doctor but it was a different doctor. I was ok with that because I love my practice; they are all so great. So I went in and explained high level what was going on with me and guess what? She, the new doctor, had three children and she had had postpartum depression with all of her three children! It was like every sentence she uttered I was like A-MEN. When she listened and shook her head I was like I got you and you got me! When she spoke the word "holistic," I was like OMG yes, yes, yes!

I am so glad to share with you what she shared with me, which are some very helpful ways to help treat postpartum depression:

- Bach's Rescue Remedy
- Hyland's Calm Forte
- Mindfulness Base Stress Reduction Training

And last but not least this web site called Postpartum Progress: http://www.postpartumprogress.com/. This site was what helped me the most from her recommendations! To be honest it wasn't until almost two months after I had seen the doctor that I felt ok. I didn't feel 100% and I wanted to talk to someone. The first thing I did was actually call a PPD hotline. I have never in my life called a hotline! Now I know why because guess what? They didn't really help! I was on the phone with them for about twenty minutes, and most of the time the woman was just researching help in my areas which I could have Googled on my own. I wanted to talk to someone then and there. Who knows? Maybe I would have gotten further if I called a suicide hotline, which is sad! At any rate, I got off the phone and remembered my doctor referring some things, mentioned above, which I had not looked into. The only thing I could really do that late at night was look at the web site so I did. I was beyond thrilled to find a forum where I could share my issues and even "talk" online with other moms who were also awake late battling the same beast as me! I am so thankful I went to my other doctor because, though I took her recommendations later, it was at the perfect moment. It was all providential in my eyes!

Aside from the fact that, thanks be to God, this woman related to me on a postpartum depression level, she knew what to test for and she did it. A full glorious work up and guess what? It all came back fine except for Vitamin D, which I was low on. That was really good to know because I never would have thought I was low on Vitamin D unless they tested it before. Looking at it now it makes total sense because I work from home, indoors, and the warmer weather had yet to come. Even though my thyroid came back okay she told me to still take the medication. I never asked why. I just trusted but knowing what a train wreck I was when I went to see her I am sure she thought best not to mess with my thyroid and give me yet another side effect to deal with. As you can see this is why it is so important to go to both doctors!

CHAPTER 7

Work Life Balance: Be Open With Your Boss

I have been blessed for I have always had good bosses. I never told my boss what I had but I was open with him. I told him I could return back to work but very slowly and I didn't know how long that would last. He was fantastic and said he would flex as long as we kept me out of the emergency room!

My co-worker was also great because she was hired to pick up where I lacked or handle my overflow. Well let's just say her cup overfloweth! She did though. She did not bother me and, even better, to this day she only supports me. She and I have been working together or connected in work or on Facebook for eight years. She knew what I had and so she was and still is always checking on me. I am blessed.

One scary thing for me is that the first week, once I got on email and was just replying to emails (not actually working or handling requests), I had to have my husband preview my emails to make sure they sounded ok. When you hit cray-cray in your mind you second guess everything so yeah, I had him double-check my emails. It gave me piece of mind. Even with my co-worker, we would be on calls with vendors and after the call I would immediately call her and ask her to please confirm that she was going to lose her mind as well on the call. And she did, and she didn't lie. She meant it. She confirmed my sanity. When you feel like you are insane, there is nothing more blissful then a confirmation that you are semi-sane.

In my case I could not cut back hours unless money was going to fall from the sky or someone was going to donate money to my "cause." So I took it slow. I don't suggest it. If you are not a masochist and if you can take time off, like Nike says JUST DO IT. Your health is the most important thing in the world (says this mom of nine only seven weeks postpartum who has been typing for twelve hours straight).

CHAPTER 8

Help and Support: When Mom Needs A Babysitter

My husband was blessed enough by his company, which allowed him to work around my schedule and my issues. So one of my biggest issues was I had to take my children to school every day at 7:30 and pick them up at 2:30. So what's the big deal? Well, it's not a big deal if your progesterone doesn't cause you dizziness to the point that you can't drive. Or if you didn't–for the first time in your life–fear things you never feared before. Fear of getting in a car and driving, fear of going to church (though you were a daily communicant), fear of seeing people at school...fear of everything.

My husband was able to drop and pick up my kids from school. This was such a blessing because he himself was a principal and a superintendent so for him not to be in his school when it opened or when it closed was huge. Talk about work and family balance!

My husband left with the six kids so I only had three kids with me...no problem, right? Wrong. Why? Because, once again – for the first time in my life – I now had a new fear, a fear which scared the bejeezus out of me: fear of being alone. Let's think about this rationally for a second. What mother does not want to be alone? It is our dream! To be alone, to pee alone, to do anything ALONE. It never happens, not even on Mother's Day when it should!

I have always wanted time alone! ALWAYS. But not this day, the day I was alone for the first time. In the very beginning of this bout with postpartum depression I did not want to be alone by myself or be alone with my children. I did it that first day. I managed to do it but only because my sister told me to call someone if I had anxiety. I did and after I talked to my mom I was fine. I did it. I managed to take care of myself and my three children. I was proud.

A few days in I had a visit from my sister, the nurse, and she launched into an action plan to have people help me. I hate to say it but over the years we have kind of drifted apart. I miss her a lot but she is very busy. However, whenever there is any medical issue whatsoever she is there. And she was. She still is. So she put together an action plan and basically set up a week of people helping me. And that is what happened. I kid you not. I had round the clock people helping me and us. It was humbling but it was needed.

I vividly remember my mom and I talking and she made some type of comment like, "you can't expect people to help when everyone is so busy with their own lives." She didn't mean it in a bad way and I understood her but I said, "Yes, you can Mom, yes you can!" Then I reminded her of how God wired her and the Mahar women (Mahar is my maiden name). I said, "I have no idea why He wired us this way but we can do a lot. It's a blessing (house is moved) and a curse (oops I got PPD in the process). But if your family and friends really love you and care about you and don't want you to die, or hey, kill your kids, they will be glad to help, trust me." I told her even in my fog, my jetlag of postpartum depression, if someone asked me for anything I would do it. That is how I am. That is how I am wired. So ladies or men out there: don't be afraid to ask for help!

For almost an entire month I had meals sent to us. They came from family, from friends, from my kid's school, from my church community. I was floored. I could not keep up. I posted and tagged people on Facebook so I would remember who did what for us when I came out of my postpartum blur.

To this day I still have not deep cleaned my house. My one girlfriend did. My babysitter has run the vacuum once a week in most of the house. My hubby does some stuff here and there. My goal has been to keep up with the laundry, fill and empty the dishwasher, and last but not least: get better. It is very humbling to look at people cleaning your house especially when my old house was always in perfect order, everything was always in its place (with the exception of toys), and Mondays were deep clean days. Talk about humble pie!

CHAPTER 9

How Do You Stop When You Can't?

I remember my sister calling me regularly at the beginning of this bout. After she checked up on me, she would always end the conversation with, "go and enjoy your family." I remember saying, "yes, I will," but also I remember thinking, "how the hell am I supposed to enjoy my family?" I mean, in my own defense, I am in a new home, with a total mess everywhere, my husband is totally sleep deprived, my children are looking at me wondering if I am going to live or not, I have a job to do, I'm nursing or pumping, oh and I have one small problem: I have postpartum depression. So yeah, her statement seemed borderline irrational thinking and trust me, I know irrational thinking! Ha!

But seriously when the fog was lifted I understood what she meant and I tried to take her advice. I let the house go, meaning I did not deep clean. Heck, I barely cleaned at all. Before the kids came home from school I made them a nice big healthy snack that was waiting for them. I played some of their favorite music. They walked in the door and were in heaven. They were probably wondering if I was June Cleaver. Who is this woman? And then I would go out and jump on the trampoline. And then I would push them on the swing. And then we would just snuggle on the couch. And, most importantly there was one tiny person who I had failed to enjoy: the newborn. I nursed him, I slept with him, I changed him, and I eventually got over the fear of bathing him but enjoying him? I had not. OMG, it slapped me in the face. Weeks had passed and I did not even enjoy the kid. So I talked to him. I looked at him. He looked at me. He smiled! It was like a ray of light. That is the day I stopped. And that was one of the best most normal days I've had.

As the months passed I followed this pattern of doing less. I did my work for my job, I straightened the house, but I relied more on the help of my children and husband. My children cleaned their rooms and then they helped me on small projects. For example, at the end of every day before dinner they helped me clean up. In the past I would have done this myself but it was exhausting and contributed to my postpartum symptoms. My husband helped me so much by simply doing whatever I didn't. He ended up mopping and vacuuming on a regular basis and sometimes I even caught him deep cleaning the bathrooms! In addition to what he did on his own he would do anything else that I asked so I tried to give him jobs which were exhausting for me. It was such a great relief to do this – in general – but also because I had always done most of the work myself. So all I can say is ask for help and just STOP and enjoy the flowers! You can stop. You must stop. You must make yourself stop. You won't regret it when you do. The dishes will always be there but the kids won't be. Enjoy your family.

CHAPTER 10

Spiritual Help And The Wild Horse That Can't Be Tamed

At the beginning of my conversion (conversion from a lukewarm Catholic to a devout one) I met a very holy priest who basically called me out and on day one of meeting me told me that I am like a wild horse that can't be tamed! I was not insulted in the least. I was actually thrilled he depicted me so accurately and from that day forward I chose him to be my spiritual director; the person I would go to confession to once a week or as needed and who would give me spiritual direction in all aspects of my life.

Years passed and my director moved to Spain. I eventually found other priests who would be my director. They have changed over the years. My last one, who has been my spiritual director for the longest time, he too had to move to Ecuador. Lucky for me he would remain my go-to director as needed via glorious Skype!

When the postpartum depression walls came crashing down around me and after I had been treated by the hospital and my OBGYN, I discovered something very scary: I couldn't pray. Think of the symptoms of postpartum depression: can't concentrate, scattered thinking, etc. So it was no wonder I could not pray. It took me seven weeks to pray a rosary. It was sad and scary. I knew God understood; I knew He was helping me and I knew that we were communicating without words but it was scary as hell. I had never not been able to pray; even when I was a teenager living a life of perpetual mortal sin, I still had prayed all the time.

Even though I couldn't pray I knew I had to reach out for help so I contacted my parish and I asked the priest if he would come and hear my confession, bring me communion and even, if possible, bring me the anointing of the sick (which was really only given in cases of death). He was at my house within an hour. I could not believe it. This just goes to show you that if you seriously ask for help your true friends and family will help you. He arrived at the house and heard my confession and I apologized to him because I wasn't sure if I was making any sense (scattered thinking) or if he could follow me. He could. He gave me communion and then he actually gave me the anointing of the sick. I had the anointing of the sick after I had the C-section with my twins. I had it once when I was in severe pain at the end of my pregnancy and now, I had it this time. This time was the most important time to have it because I literally felt like I was going to die inside and out. It is a feeling so very hard to articulate but maybe one that, if you have postpartum depression and you are reading this, you will understand.

This priest, Father James, came not only that time but a few other times. See I hadn't left the house, so as to recuperate and also because I had a fear of everything. That priest came, he helped me, and he would have kept coming no matter how long I had asked him.

Eventually I was able to go back to church and I have to say it was very hard for me. I had major anxiety about going because that is where it all came crashing down on me. So the first time I went to church I went to a different one. I didn't go in the main church because I was afraid of becoming over-stimulated. I stayed in the library but I was there and could hear the whole Mass. Eventually I made it back to my parish and though it was hard at first, it was good to be back. I wanted to be normal again so I had to get back in the saddle and just go there!

Once I arrived to the point where I found myself feeling normal again my prayer life began to change. Because I had experienced such darkness, I was able to appreciate the light so much more. In that regard though the wave of postpartum depression was very difficult I do think that because of it now my spiritual life is better. It is hard to see the good through the bad. It is hard to know why this is happening to us but eventually you reach an awakening and you see how what has occurred can help you and more importantly help others. Because of this change in my personal spiritual life when I see a momma struggling with what I believe is postpartum depression I reach out immediately. Things happen for a reason.

We may not always understand why but if your situation can help someone or even save their life then you just took all the bad and gave it purpose.

You would be surprised at how many women are struggling out there without anyone noticing or asking about them. I find great joy and even a spiritual consolation in knowing that I may be able to help them with my story.

CHAPTER 11

Don't Take Anything For Granted

I have said several times that postpartum depression for me has been a blessing and a curse. It is a curse for the obvious reasons. Who the hell wants anxiety, depression, panic attacks, etc.? The blessings are numerous for me. For one, with my first bout of it I learned to appreciate those in my life who do suffer from very serious panic and/or anxiety attacks. I never fully understood it until I had one. Now I can relate to those people.

I will never forget, after I recognized the bout the first time, I had gone to church and a person who suffered from mental illness came up to me. She had always come up to me and since she suffers from mental illness I never knew what I was going to get from her. One day she'd call me slut and the next day she'd be my best friend. I never minded her until I had postpartum depression and she came up and started rambling to me. I just kept thinking in my head, "please make her stop because right now my head is her vocals. My head won't stop and she won't stop so now it is like an explosion in and out of my head of crazies: she and me." I let her finish and then left the church. I didn't even stay for that daily Mass because she overwhelmed me. But now, when I see a person who struggles from mental illness I embrace them because this, what I have, is a mental illness. Thank God it can be PREVENTABLE (rule number one: don't be a masochist) and it can be treated with or without meds (rule number two: go to your doctors!).

Before this bout with postpartum depression I feel as if I took so much for granted. I had so much anxiety about driving. Driving? Driving. When you are overwhelmed in your head, when you are sleep deprived for weeks, when you are just starting hormone therapy or medicine, it takes a while to have everything sync up. So for me there was no way I could operate a vehicle. Weeks later after I had been treated, I learned the hard way that though I want to get my jam on in the car I couldn't. I had put on a newly released album and I was loving it. The next thing I knew I was about to be hit by a car because when I hit the stop sign I looked right but not left. As I saw the car coming I froze literally. That is not ok. And I felt like either my foot finally caught up with my body or my guardian angel pressed the pedal to the metal and got me out of that bind. Note to self: don't try to drive and jam! You are not dizzy but you clearly can't walk and chew gum at the same time – at least not yet!

Doing the normal things I did before: enjoying a cup of coffee, going out, pushing a vacuum in one room (let alone the house), sweeping the kitchen, wiping down the counters in the kitchen. Those little things that we take for granted every day, I hope to never ever take for granted again. I couldn't do these things before. I had to watch hopelessly in a chair while someone else cleaned my whole house. I was envious. I thought I would never be able to do so many things again for myself or for my family.

And then, last but not least, there is the blessing of this, my dream, my book. After I had my kids, I always wanted to be an author. I started my book almost three years ago. And yet, postpartum depression this time around gave me such an inspiration to be the voice to it. No, to be the blaring bullhorn pain in the butt mom that no one can stand but friend nonetheless. This book is a blessing to me if to no one else because it brought me my dreams and it only took a few days alone (and a lot of drive) to do it.

CHAPTER 12

Baby Steps

Did you ever see the movie What About Bob? It's pretty hilarious. In short Bob is a patient and he suffers from not wanting to touch anything without gloves. His doctor advises him to take baby steps. Baby steps to the door, baby steps to open the door, baby steps to close the door. You get the idea.

This movie and concept helped me so much because that is how I tackled the first few days without help. I had been afraid to touch the baby, hold the baby... This was in the very beginning. I especially did not want to bathe the baby. When the baby slept with me I would wake up every other minute to make sure he was breathing. So I began to take baby steps to doing things and it worked out great for me.

There is something very strange about this illness when you are in it and not on medication. It can be like an out of body experience. It is very hard to articulate it but I can try. There were moments in the very beginning where I felt like time literally stood still. It didn't move. The clock didn't budge. And then there were moments where everything would fly by. For example, I basically wrote this book in one seven hour sitting and it felt like a minute. Or, for example, the first time I went shopping with my daughter. I was standing in the line at Wal-Mart to do some returns. It was totally unnecessary but since I do the accounting in my family I wanted my cash back! I remember being in the line and it was as if I could read lips. I watched people around me and I took in my surroundings like never before. It is a surreal and scary experience. It just feels like an out of body experience; there is no other way to explain it. I am only comforted in knowing that others do share this crazy side effect, which does go away.

For me, as the wave of postpartum depression continued on and I began to learn how to ride it, baby steps were always a part of the balancing act. It could be something as simple as telling myself today I am only going to do this one thing – whatever it was. In the very beginning it could have been, "I am only going to focus on baby." In the middle it could have been, "today I am going to clean the kitchen." In the end it could have been, "today I am going to clean the house." As with any Fitbit, little steps add up! So just try to continually take baby steps in all you do and it will help you little by little to get back to whatever your normal is!

CHAPTER 13

Face Your Fears

When I started coming to, as you might say, from the postpartum depression I knew that the only way I could get better was if I faced my fears. And so I did. The first thing I did was I decided to drive two miles away. I know, two miles may seem like a joke to you but for me, who was ridden with fear and anxiety, two miles was like a road trip to Rome. It felt almost impossible. I got in the car and though I didn't pray because it was still hard to pray, I made the sign of the cross and off I went. I made sure to focus like never before. Be overly cautious, I thought. People behind me probably thought I was an old lady because when I hit major intersections I waited for everyone – even a duck – to cross over to the other lane. If I was going to do this I was going to be cautious. And I did it. I came back to my driveway with such a great sense of relief. I went live on Facebook, which I had rarely done, and I shared my joy.

My next attempt at facing my fears was going to pick up my kids at school with my husband. He drove and we purposely got there late so that I would not have to see too many people. I remember running into one woman who asked me how I was - knowing that I had postpartum depression and it was almost as if she thought I was completely over it. I chuckled inside thinking, baby I am seriously going to have to watch this very closely for a year or more. Because people don't understand postpartum depression or because they toss it to the side, I just let it roll off me (though I was thinking, when this is done I need to be a bullhorn for this illness which has basically taken over my life). When my kids came running out to me and saw me there it was sheer bliss. For three weeks I had not picked up my kids. Up until the baby was born I was the only one really to do it so this moment was not only huge for them but for me too.

From there we went to something that I do twice every year: I went to a major consignment sale! My dear friend Linda, who ran the sale, let me in before anyone so I could shop. I think within one hour I had spent $400, the most I had ever spent. I definitely was not thinking clearly but I don't regret it. Everything I got was for my kids and mostly for Christmas, which was a mere six months away! It was so great to make it to that sale. I didn't think I would but I did it.

One of the next fears I faced was your regular stuff: going grocery shopping, doing the loop as I call it (dollar store, Wal-Mart, Sam's club, etc.). I also went out for a girl's night to someone's house. I will be honest and say that that was the night that I felt like I had to take a Xanax but I didn't. I worked through the feelings and thoughts on my own while all the ladies sat around me. I was proud not only that I got out but that I worked through it and did not have to take a Xanax.

So it was facing my fears, one at a time, that gave me some sanity, some stability. It took weeks to get there but hey, who cares if it takes months to get there so long as you get there. So face your fears, you won't regret it!

CHAPTER 14

Go Off The Grid and Just Say No!

When I discovered I had postpartum depression, the first thing to go was as much technology as possible. I am a huge Facebook person. I am huge news person. I love to know what is going on all over the world and locally. But I just could not. It was too much stimulation to me and too much of a distraction to me. So the first thing I did was announce on Facebook that I was going to be M.I.A. And I did. I didn't say why. I did not read the news, I did not text much, and I did not email much, nothing. And that was huge for me personally. The same with the TV, etc. Once we got the kids off to school, it was no iPads for the little ones, no computer, no TV. All of that was just extra noise and keep in mind, I had to battle with the noise in my head, that mind racing, etc. So I had to remove any other noise and it worked wonders for me.

The other thing that I have to say is just say no to anything and anyone. I was blessed in that not many people ask me to do things because I have so many children but I will give you an example of how I had to say no! Because we are a big family people always want to give me hand-me-downs. People knew I had postpartum depression, people knew I had just moved into a new house and was in a huge war zone with things all over the place and yet these beloved people -who had every good intention- would drop off bags and bags and bags of kids' clothes to me! I remember one day all my sister did the entire day was sort those bags by gender and size. I kept thinking she could have helped me so much by doing something else that really needed to be done! So I went onto my Facebook and I nicely told everyone that while I would forever be happy to take their "crap" as they called it off their hands I just asked for them to not do it now. And luckily no one got offended and they did stop and they resumed after I felt better!

The other funny thing that happened unintentionally for me is that I became a Mark Zuckerberg (the owner of Facebook) without intending to be! I had discovered that I was wearing the same exact outfit for like weeks: long black t-shirt with gray yoga pants. I did not do it intentionally. It just kind of happened. Because I had two of the same outfit and because I do laundry every day it was just easier for me to grab the same outfit. I had chuckled to myself when I noticed it and remembered that I had seen this video on Facebook where Mark had explained why he wears the same outfit every day: gray t-shirt, jeans and a black hoodie. He said it was one less decision to have to make in the morning! By having the same outfit he could just get out of the shower and go. Genius! And in my case, for postpartum depression this was ideal because there were so many decisions to make with the house that it is true; to have one less thing to think about was so key.

The other thing I can suggest, and this is coming from an organized hoarder, is to be a minimalist. When we moved into the house we put everything in the garage and we worked from there. We only moved things into the house that we absolutely needed. Well guess what? We discovered that we don't really need a lot and that too much stuff is just more clutter and more work. When you have clutter of the mind with postpartum depression, to have less physical clutter can help you mentally. Ah, 'tis true trust me! So here I am months later in the house and the garage is still full. 75% of the kids' toys are hidden. Do I need that stuff? Do they? No. So my goal is to have a gigantic garage sale and free myself from that which I do not need and which causes me more work and more stress!

CHAPTER 15

Irrational Thinking, Dangerous Objects, and The Goldfish That Had To Go

Triggers are very important to recognize because if you are treating yourself or being treated holistically or via hormone therapy, if you attack your trigger at its root and pull it then you can prevent potential setbacks and, even worse, disasters.

It is so scary to me that dangerous objects never bothered me with my first bout of postpartum depression or ever. However this time I just remember thinking to myself, "should I have my husband lock up the razors, the knives, the safety pins, the iron, the flat iron, and all those things that I could hurt myself with?" When I was younger I cut myself but more for attention. I had suicidal thoughts and tendencies I never told my family about it but I wrote about it in a journal. This is why I am all for reading your kids' journal, texts, etc. My friends knew about it at that time but cutting yourself was the thing to do. I still have scars and I hate them because they remind me of really bad toxic relationships with both friends and boyfriends. To be honest, looking back I am wondering if the suicidal thoughts were just for attention amongst my friends. Maybe.

At any rate, I never had my husband do anything with the dangerous objects because I felt that I could control my thoughts or my actions on those thoughts unlike people who have postpartum psychosis. Brooke Shields shared her stories of wanting to drive off the road with her child. Yeah, I had that. I also had thoughts like what if I take my baby, who was in his lamb rocker, and just drop the lamb rocker over the top of stairs but in a gentle way. A totally insane fleeting thought but an example of why one needs to be treated. And keep in mind one can be treated either with or without medication and not only still have these thoughts but have them intensify to the point where one acts on them. Welcome to postpartum depression: the illness that, if discussed as it should be, could save a lot of moms' lives, a lot of kids' lives, and a lot of heartache and pain for all involved but no, we shoebox the illness because it makes us effin' uncomfortable. We can talk about animal rights and the like 'til thy kingdom come but talk about a life or death illness in the world and no, shoebox that baby and put a freaking bow on it. Sad.

One night when I was overloaded with my job (I had doubled my workload that week working 40 hours) and my husband was late, I looked at the carnival goldfish. As a backdrop, one year ago my kids walked in with a carnival goldfish and I was so mad. We had been through this before. We had fish and they died and I had to deal with the drama. No more pets. Some people have pets, some people have children, and some people have both. Though I am a masochist, in the case of pets I am not. My children are enough work for me; I do not need pets. So I figured this fish would die soon. It did not.

We took care of it for almost a year. I actually became friends with it. Then carnival comes up again and I forgot to warn them not to get a fish and what do they show up with? A fish. I was like no. All the kids were so happy because the other fish had a friend. So we put the fish in with the other fish and they were ok for a few days. Then the big fish started freaking out. I thought he was chasing the fish because he was trying to eat it. I fed him and all was ok. Then I thought maybe they are the opposite sex and one is trying to attack the other and make babies because come on, only we would have a fish that would have a million babies, right? Probably my luck. Then he just kept freaking out and I didn't know why. Then the next day my kid says the big fish is dead. What? Oh boy was I mad. You have to be kidding me. Then I recalled someone on my blog telling me that the new one could get the other one sick. That is what happened: the new fish - that was immediately named Jaws- got the other one sick. I was actually mad. I mourned the fish but not a typical mourning. We had a ceremony and my husband had to try hard not to laugh at the Catholic prayers for the ceremony. I am sorry; I am just very detached from the pet thing, clearly. So we bury the fish and at that point I am hoping and praying the other fish dies. Not only didn't I want the fish, I didn't want the work and I was resentful that the fish killed the other fish. He took away the "person" I talked to in the middle of the night. He took away the "person" that mimicked me. I would run around my house like a chicken with its head cut off and so did he in the tank, pacing viciously back and forth. I would actually miss the first fish. So on this night when I was overworked (trigger) and done in and waiting for my husband who was late I walked over and noticed that the fish was floating to the top. That is a telltale sign that he is dying. I have seen it multiple times before and I knew that this was the end, my friend. So, in my unclear thinking I decided I would put the fish out of its misery. I would go old school and flush the fish down the toilet even though I knew that was not good for him. I was not in my right mind so forgive me. Someone, something had to go and it was Jaws. So after the thought I wasted no time. I scooped up the fish and made sure no one saw me and I tossed him down the toilet, saying my peace to him, nicely wishing him well to fish heaven and I did it. I flushed. He went down. I saw him go down. I went to bed after my hubby arrived with no regrets and not cleaning the tank knowing that no one would probably notice for weeks that he was gone because who takes care of the fish despite the chore chart? Moi. Well wouldn't you know it, an hour later my husband went to use the bathroom and he saw the fish swimming around in the toilet and almost died. The kids ran in and my son literally rescued it with his bare hands. Jaws has some balls clearly. That friggin' fish swam like Nemo damn it. Only me. So I denied anything to my kids and confessed to my husband. I warned the kids because the toilet water was different that he may not live and I warned him he was floating to the top anyways. Weeks later the damn fish not only lives but he thrives. What have I gathered from this experience? That even if I wanted to be a mass murderer I couldn't actually kill a fly because I am clearly meant to live with as many babies and a fish (or two) as possible. Only me. I can't make this stuff up. Moral of this story: during postpartum depression do not ever act on your feelings and irrational thoughts! Oh, and don't get a pet!

CHAPTER 16

Who's That In The Mirror? Will I Ever Be Normal Again?

One thing that happened to me right away when I had this bout of postpartum depression is that I could not look at myself in the mirror. It scared the crap out of me. It goes back to the out-of-body experience. If I caught a glance of myself in the mirror it was like I was outside by body looking at me and I did not recognize me. At first it was just my face. That was not me. I looked sad but I wasn't. I was frustrated because this happened. I was frustrated because I thought I caused it. I was frustrated because I do not ask for help ever except for paid help and everyone was helping me for free. I was frustrated because I did not think this would ever end. I just wanted to be in my body, be normal, and recognize myself in the mirror.

Then something scary and yet glorious at the same time happened; one day I looked in the mirror and I noticed something. I was skinnier like a lot skinnier. I weighed myself. In two weeks of giving birth I had lost like almost thirty pounds and let me clarify something: when I left the hospital I had an 8 lb 12 oz pound baby but lost 7 pounds so yeah, this was huge for me on several levels.

My whole life I have been very conscious of my body and my weight. Later in life I became conscious of my health and what I ate. I gained 55 pounds with my first baby. I lost 20 after him and then got pregnant and since then I have never gotten back to my first pregnancy weight. I have dieted and exercised all these years in the hopes of losing the weight but I have only lost the new baby weight and have basically been carrying around 45-50 extra pounds for all these years. So for me to drop 30 pounds in two weeks and not know it or recognize it was insane. I was sad and thrilled at the same time. I was sad because my milk supply was down. I was sad because my husband slept with the baby downstairs so I could sleep but as the experts say, the more you sleep the more you lose, and clearly that was true! I was sad because I know dieting so I was like, what happens when I get my appetite back? See I had no appetite. To have four crackers was like having a hamburger with cheese, side of fries and a milkshake. I just couldn't. I still can't. And yet I was thrilled because finally I weighed the lowest I had in eight or more years! Glory!

I was also thrilled because since I hadn't done much, since I slept lot, since I was on progesterone and Xanax as needed I did not have anxiety so guess what? The habit I had for oh say 35 years of biting my nails? It ceased. And on one of the days that I woke up from postpartum depression I discovered not only did I have nails but I had beautiful, long, healthy nails! I was floored. I have had tips to hide the nail biting. I have bought dollar store kits but this? Wow this was freaking authentic! I was elated! And I never touched my nails again until much later when I started feeling better.

You talk about being normal and when will you be normal again? Who the heck knows? I hate so much of this. I hate not taking care of the/my/our baby at night but when I do it sets me back. I hate that my husband does not sleep with me. I used to shun it when people would say they slept in two rooms. Yeah, now I am blowing every effin' thing out the window. I suck. I judged. And now, I am in it. Am I in it to win it? Hell yes so guess what, my hubby sleeps on the couch. Probably will for like ever. I even prayed for a pet! I don't believe in pet heaven but hell, I prayed for a pet because you know what, when you have this illness anything goes. I have done the unthinkable in my mind but you know what, it helped me cope, get by, so I would do it all again. Even my kids could not believe that I would let them purposely get dirty and stay dirty for fun. Who are you, Mom? But it caused me more stress to fight with them than to just let them get dirty. So, yeah anything goes when you have postpartum depression!

I remember my kids looking at me at the beginning of this second bout. They did not even notice the first bout because super mom hid it from them and coped with it alone in the darkness of the night. But this time around everything was different. When the police came to our new house the kids missed it because they were in their new big rooms. They missed Mom going out on a stretcher. I was almost annoyed like can't you witness my sickness?

But later they did, oh they did. In the weeks following my trip to the emergency room there were times you could see my children look at me and they knew that something was very wrong with Mommy. They would look at me and honestly not know if they should smile, laugh, or cry. "Is she ok? Is she being funny because she's normal? Is she being funny because she's gone crazy? She's crying; I'm sad." And when I would cry in front of them or tell them I would be ok but I was not, they would embrace me. They actually took care of me.

Many weeks in to the second bout, this bout, my beloved second born celebrated his first Holy Communion. The celebration of any sacrament is always a huge day for us. So I ran around ragged all morning (which in postpartum diagnosis I should not have). I arrived at the church in time and then I had to sit there in the place that was my best place before but the place where it all came crashing down on me and so now it was the worst place. I sat there for an hour and a half and it was torture. I hated sitting up front; I was anxious but in masochistic terms it is the best spot to view the communion and take the best pictures. So I held the spot knowing that I could not ever sit there during the ceremony. It was so sad. My son did not understand why the whole entourage would be there but not me. I said, as an excuse, "I have the twins; we need to be in the cry room." (I only brought the twins so that I could have a reason for him and all family and friends to know why I was going to be in the cry room). But I assured him I saw it all from the back and took a video (which I did) but it was not the same. When will I be normal enough to sit in a church and not a foyer or a cry room? When will I be me again? Damn it! It is not fair to my husband, to my kids and to me! But, if you are experiencing these feelings, not to worry (!) for normalcy will return to you just as it did to me!

CHAPTER 17

Do You All.The.Time.

I hope you don't take this title the wrong way! But this is the truth, when you have severe postpartum depression you need to take care of yourself. You need to let people take care of you, even if it is hard. And basically you have to do you like all the time. Does this mean that you do nothing for no one else? Heck no. Because for me, in my case, to be able to help my husband, my kids, my friends and family gave me a sense of normalcy. That is not what I mean. I mean don't feel bad for focusing on yourself and getting better.

Everyone who knows me knows that my husband and I go out alone once a month at a minimum. If we can go out more, we do. It all comes down to money. But that time is key for our marriage and so it is something that we always do. That was the same during my postpartum depression. I remember being so happy because we were going to go out one night. But guess what happened? I did not sleep well the night before so I woke up feeling set back and I knew that if I would go out it would just push me further backwards; it would be good for the postpartum depression (as far as getting out) but not for me. So I canceled but it was all right because a mere week later we went out and had the best date night ever!

Because I am trying to live holistically, I firmly believe in massage therapy. I have gotten it regularly for years. Some people may do other things or take other medications but my thing is massage therapy. So after I started resuming normal activities I went and got a massage and it felt so great and to be honest that night of sleep was the best one I had had since the onset of my postpartum depression.

I also took some time with my daughters and went and got a pedicure and a manicure. I had never ever in my life had a manicure because I had never had nails. You would think that since I had bitten my nails all my life and since one of the major symptoms I was experiencing was anxiety you would think I would have had even smaller nails but I didn't because nothing makes any freaking sense when you have this illness. I have no idea why I had not bitten my nails but now that I had gotten a manicure and had seen how pretty my nails were I vowed never to bite them again!

Since we had moved into the new house and we had this gigantic Jacuzzi tub, which could fit both my husband and me in it (he is 6'4),I decided to take daily baths. For maybe ten years of our marriage I had taken five baths. I never had time. No, I never made the time. Well now I was making the time. What did it take anyway? A sheer thirty minutes extra per day? It seems so minimal but when you are a mom who never stops, thirty minutes seems like a day. Those baths relaxed me and made my sleeping so much better.

I went out for girl's night with my best friend. She was always so busy and it was very hard to get together but one day I just flat out told her: I need to talk to you, I need to see you, and like a best friend does, she dropped everything and we went out that night.

So yeah, do you as much as you can and it will help you get back to normalcy. It will help you to be a better mom, a better wife, and a happier, healthier person!

CHAPTER 18

Never Run Out of Wine. Like EVER. & Self-Medicating

I always say some people like drugs, some people like prescription drugs and then some people like me like wine. Oh yes, may the wine never run out! May it always be overflowing in my home! I am sorry to say it but it is true. For as long as I can remember I have been a wino. Ha! It takes the edge off for me; it helps me get to sleep, etc. That is one reason why I do not like to take prescription drugs because most of them you cannot drink with. That is another reason why I never want to take the Xanax and if I have to I am sure to ask my sister if it is ok, meaning one day at lunch I had a glass of wine and then five hours or more later I had a panic attack and took a Xanax and freaked out. I called my sister and she said it was ok because of the time lapse. Whew. Thank goodness I can take progesterone and still have my wine! I will say though that if you Google progesterone you will see that it is says something about the liver (if you have liver problems you shouldn't take it). I don't have liver problems but I do love my wine so to balance it out I personally take the supplement milk thistle, which is an aid for the liver. I swear by it. A year or so prior to getting pregnant I had a spot on my liver that was due to fatty acid (being obese). So I took milk thistle and when I went for a follow-up the spot was completely gone from my liver! So yeah, take your milk thistle if you are like me!

One thing I had to learn the hard way is, no matter what you think, do not self-medicate. When my doctor prescribed progesterone he told me that I could take two to four pills a day. So at first I did four a day. Then a week later, after feeling good I cut back to two a day without telling him. Then a few days later I cut back to one pill a day. Ok, so one pill a day was never an option right? So dumb me, one day after Aunt Flow (my menstrual cycle) returned in all of her glory, I found myself acting irrational and having a panic attack. I was also dizzy. I know you get dizzy from taking the pills but this was different. I honestly felt like I had the day it all came crashing down on me in the church. I thought to myself in the car, oh no, is it the progesterone? And I had remembered that my Creighton person had said to watch out for when I got my period while having postpartum depression. I paged my doctor in the hospital and sure enough he told me it was that I had cut back too much on my progesterone and that is what was causing all of those symptoms including the different dizziness. I learned the hard way but immediately he said back to four pills a day and since then I have never even attempted to cut back. So moral of the story is save yourself the trouble and don't self-medicate!

CHAPTER 19

Charting Hell

For those of you who have never attempted to do Natural Family Planning or The Creighton Method let me start by explaining that both methods require that you actually use a chart to record the signs of fertility. Many people think that the only reason to try these methods is to avoid pregnancy or achieve pregnancy and while that is true there are so many more advantages to these methods. For example, by simply recording the signs of your body one can notice gynecological problems such as ovarian cancer. Working with a certified Creighton instructor and your OBGYN (especially if he or she knows Creighton) could literally save your life!

I will be honest and say that no matter what I did I could not get either of these methods down pat - clearly - and that is precisely why we have so many children back-to-back. For us, it is not about taking birth control, for that is against our religion and we take that very seriously. Additionally and very unfortunately when I was younger (way before I met my husband) I took birth control. I took the pill and Depo-Provera. I was on them for years and now looking back I wonder what the heck they did to my body besides the obvious, which for me was major weight gain. So because I try to live in a holistic manner, even if I did not practice my faith so seriously, I would not be on birth control ever again.

We were blessed in that after the birth of my eighth child I did figure it out! It was just like the scene of the movie My Fair Lady, By Golly I think she's got it! I took extreme measures to master the chart and my signs of fertility. I researched more than just what I was doing, which was Creighton at the time. I did several things which confirmed my cycles and the accuracy of my fertility. I would share it here but quite honestly I want to write a book about it!

So some of you may be wondering, well if you got it down pat, how did number nine come about? First let me explain that we are always open to life. There is always a risk of getting pregnant just like with any birth control; nothing is 100% effective. While some saintly people can abstain for extremely long periods of time we cannot! Ha! So we were practicing Creighton and we were away for our anniversary; the best anniversary trip we ever had and we knew that there was like a 5% chance that we could become pregnant and we agreed to take that chance. We were, however, a little floored when we saw that 5% chance did happen. Number nine, Philip, was the first one who was ever conceived in such a small window. But, I guess as my friends joke and say, you could sneeze on me and I would get pregnant! It is a blessing and a curse. And though I joke about it my heart always aches severely for those women who can't get pregnant or as easily as I can.

But I digress; back to the sacred chart. I knew from the week of the big house move that I had likely screwed my cycle up. Normally the return of my cycle would be when I started weaning the baby from nursing. In this case I was already giving the baby more bottles and a pacifier, both of which are not good for my cycle. So I had a feeling I was going to see Aunt Flow very soon. When I ended up in the emergency room I knew I was royally screwed for lack of better words. I knew that the stress my body had endured was really bad for my cycle. As the fog of postpartum depression set in week after week and day after day, my milk supply diminished. I knew the end was near. I also knew that taking progesterone would likely bring my cycle back on. And then one day, out of nowhere, there was Aunt Flow! My period was back and it was a completely normal cycle for me. The timing was good only in that I had just started charting a few days before.

In one way I was happy that my cycle was back. I know you probably think I am nuts! But when you chart, having your cycle back means you can chart effectively so as not to get pregnant (or, if you are on the other side, to achieve pregnancy). After a few days of my period I noticed I was spotting. What the heck? In all of my life I have never spotted outside of pregnancy. I had almost thought I was getting a second period. That lasted a few days and then nothing for five days and then alas, back to spotting again. This went on for several weeks in the same pattern. It was totally freaking me out because when you look in the Creighton book it can only mean a few things: low progesterone (I was on progesterone!), menopause (at age 39?), or something serious like cancer!

The good news was I was just due for my six-week postpartum visit with my doctor. I showed him my chart and he told me not to worry. He said it could be stress as well. He offered to do an ultrasound and I agreed. Well lo and behold we found out what it was: leftover membranes from the placenta. Apparently a very small amount did not make its way out and that was causing the spotting.

I was relieved to know what it was. Now it was just a matter of waiting it out (meaning waiting for it to pass) or to have it removed by the doctor. I chose to wait it out now that I knew what it was. If I were to compare my old charts to my new chart I would have said I was not the same person and I honestly attribute that to the postpartum depression. Aside from this leftover membrane, I think taking the progesterone and my postpartum depression were skewing my chart. My biomarkers (the signs that we look for like mucus) were completely different and thus put me in charting hell. I was afraid to get pregnant, very afraid. But I will tell you what, as crazy as it sounds I was not so much afraid to get pregnant in general but afraid of what everyone would think if I got pregnant that soon. People would naturally assume we wanted to be pregnant not knowing that I was in charting hell.

Eventually I am very happy to say that my chart leveled out but I have to say I completely attribute it to postpartum depression. Yes, I was taking progesterone but my chart did not get completely normal until I was off progesterone. Did the progesterone help? Absolutely. I believe it helped my moods as well as kick start my body back into its normal progesterone levels. However, I do think that the depression, the stress, the anxiety, the insomnia, that is what skewed my chart. I think that the progesterone changed my biomarkers but now I know what to look for should I be on it again. It is amazing to me how much can affect our cycles. I never thought I would say I was happy to see Aunt Flow or positive ovulation tests, but I really was because that meant I was getting back to me, to normal. During the wave of postpartum depression, the greatest feeling is coming up from under water and seeing the shore and know that at least you have made it!

CHAPTER 20

What's Your Trigger? Don't Pull it! Listen To Your Body; It Speaks!

I remember a few days into being alone I had a cup of coffee. Within a few sips of the coffee (which, if for Beyoncé, Girls Run The World, coffee has run my world since I was like ten. Yes ten, my parents rocked!) I realized I was getting anxious. OMG. No, heck to the no! Coffee was my first trigger. In fact any caffeine was. So I stopped. I did not have any caffeine. I switched to tea (insert finger in mouth and proceed to gag). Who the hell wants tea after a night of sleep deprivation? Not me. I want an IV of coffee or a caffeine patch from whatever Disney movie that is from. So after a week of the same darn tea I switched and sure enough within one third of a cup of drinking it I became panicky. My nurse friend arrived to my house and I had her go through the garbage to see if there was caffeine in the tea. Sure enough there was. Thanks a lot God. You take away everything from me with this illness. You can't even leave me that which allows me to function? My beloved espresso or any even crappy caffeine?! As Saint Teresa of Avila said after getting knocked off her horse and thrown in the mud, "If this is how you treat your friends Lord it's no wonder you have so few!" Amen, sista (and Saint). Joking aside, for almost two months I went without a lot of caffeine. To be honest, as much as I love coffee, I do not crave it physically. I crave it mentally because it was my BFF for so long.

The next trigger was lack of sleep, clearly. I wanted to nurse my baby. I wanted to snuggle with my husband. I wanted to co-sleep. But every time I tried, the next day I woke up feeling off, anxious and jet lagged to the point where I was debating taking a Xanax. So unfortunately my milk supply diminished and my hubby was sleeping on the couch and for the first time ever, he was taking the baby all night. But it saved me. I am not ready yet to go back to my normal schedule. I may never be but I am going to hold on to hope that I will. One thing I have learned to do is that if I can't rest or shut my mind off, I lay down for one hour every day at naptime. I just rest even if I do not sleep. It helps a lot. I also go to bed super early. After we eat as a family I go to bed if I can. I don't care if it is five, six, or seven. If I go to bed and sleep five hours and wake up at midnight I'll take it because hey I wake up to silence and well, you know silence is golden! But if I struggle with going back to sleep I just take a melatonin and within an hour I am back into a deep sleep. Melatonin has saved me over the years. There are side effects: weight gain, crossing into the milk and making baby tired and it can mess with your cycles. Google that one. That's an OK one to Google. But in that way I am in bed some nights for twelve hours and it is great for the mind, body, and soul even if I am not actually sleeping twelve hours. If I do not take a melatonin my husband will pray over me and that too puts me back to sleep like a baby! Scout's honor, try it!

The other trigger that I noticed for me is stressful situations and confrontations. I had a really bad situation with a few family members. It was really bad. It caused fights with my husband. I lost my peace. I had a setback. I took a Xanax because it was too much for me. A total of four Xanax over seven weeks. You would think I overdosed but for me, I do not like any medication if I do not have to do it. So now I try to avoid any confrontations or stressful situations.

One thing that was not a trigger but was just too much stimulation and too overwhelming for me was Facebook, email, and social media. Basically all technology. I wanted quiet. I did not want the TV on. I did not want to hear those same Minecraft guys' voices. I was ready to break the TV as their voices pushed me to the edge. So I told everyone, me who Facebooks my life away, I was going to be M.I.A. on Facebook. And I did. The only thing I really did for a while was I hashtagged my journey through postpartum depression so I could go back and see myself and see the transformations, the setbacks, etc. It helped me write this book. I would have forgotten a lot had I not posted a lot. But that was it; I would go on, post and leave.

CHAPTER 21

Oh Crap! Now I'm depressed!

Several weeks have passed since I wrote the majority of this book. In that timeframe I have been riding the many waves of postpartum depression. There were days that I felt almost 90% normal only to have something happen to set me back.

One of the things that I did not expect at all was to be depressed! I had some of what I call self-inflicted depression growing up. I call it that because I dated or fell for the wrong guys and either I wasted years trying to get them to date me or I wasted years in a bad relationship. Because of my choices I ended up depressed at times. The same later in my adult life: I made some poor decisions and I ended up somewhat depressed. However, as an adult I was able to overcome it easily and without medications. I basically threw myself into my work and that solved my problem!

So you could imagine my shock when, after having gone maybe eleven years without being depressed, one day I wake up depressed! In my case I was depressed because my body was not normalizing in that my cycles were playing games with me. I thought I had my period and maybe I did but then it disappeared for months. Some of the biomarkers in my body were returning and that made me very happy but when I was getting negatives on the ovulation tests and I was not getting a period I was wondering what was wrong with me! I took pregnancy tests and they were negative. What the hell did I do to my body? What was happening inside?

I called my doctor and he agreed to do all types of hormone tests. That was really the last straw because we knew why I was spotting, and we also knew that all of my other tests had come back normal except for a lack of vitamin D. I nearly died the day he called me and told me that according to the results of the tests I was infertile! Can you imagine? He told me that I should look to my family history in regards to menopause. He also said that we know that I am normally very fertile so he did think the results were strange but he also did not think that I was in menopause. I pushed a little further and requested a FSH hormonal test to see if in fact my body was in menopause. I was very happy to hear that I was not, yet I was still confused.

This whole conversation in union with my body being so weird basically made me depressed. I was depressed because if I was not menopausal what was wrong with me? Did I stress my body out so much that it would takes months on end to get back to normal? Was I menopausal? If I was, that really depressed me. It is horrible to say but it is the truth in that so many times in my marriage I have prayed to be infertile. I was stressed out, overwhelmed and just did not want any more kids. I thought maybe I will have to have a hysterectomy after birth and I thought that it would be a dream. I know, totally crazy especially to women who can't get pregnant but for me, I was perpetually pregnant and so yes, I wanted a break, a long break or to be totally done. However, when I thought that I could not have any more children alas I became depressed. Now that my body was not ovulating I was depressed. Now that I was without a period I felt less of a woman and that made me depressed.

There was a good week or so when, after getting the kids to school, I kinda just laid on the sofa and lived in that depressing moment for a long time. I didn't want to take medication and I knew it would pass but I actually wanted to live in that depressing moment for some odd reason. Eventually I got to the point where I realized, like always, I was not in charge of my fertility so I just had to ride that wave out. And I am. There I was for weeks with my body screwed up. I couldn't chart properly and even if I had a sex drive (which I didn't because for some women the first thing to go in postpartum depression is a sex drive) I wouldn't want my husband to come near me because I was and am still afraid to get pregnant. My hope was that as time healed me it would heal my body and she would return to doing what she was supposed to: ovulating even if I never get pregnant again. It is one thing to know that you are going into menopause but it's another thing to not know what your body is up to. I am a 39-year-old woman with symptoms of someone in her mid 50s; it just ain't right!

CHAPTER 22

Who's talking about Postpartum Depression? No one, that's who.

I think the most "depressing" part of postpartum depression for me is that no one talks about it. Sure, you hear about it in the hospital right after you give birth but that is pretty much it. And I honestly hate that because for the love of God you just had a baby; your body is out of whack. How the heck can you possibly know if you have postpartum depression? I didn't. Or what happens when you go home and you experience all these symptoms and you roll with it or think it is normal? It's not normal and it should be treated but how do you know that?

This is one reason why I wrote this book. I am not doing it to be famous. I am not doing it for the money (though money is always needed in a big family and it would be nice!). No, I am doing it to get the word out. Finally you see some celebrities talking about this illness openly. I am so happy about that. But what about the doctors? The hospitals? The medical community at large? What about your neighbor, your friend? No one talks about it. There is a stigma to postpartum depression and unless you have gone through it you have no idea how serious it is.

If, as Beyoncé says, Girls Run The World what would happen if every girl who actually got pregnant and every girl actually had postpartum depression and what if every girl did not get treated for it and what if every girl killed themselves and their child or children because of the irrational thinking of postpartum depression? I'll tell you what would happen: the entire effin' world would end. Period. Because newsflash, no matter how great science is, you need a woman to have children and keep the world population rising. So yeah, it's kind of important to talk about this even if no one else is.

One thing that really frustrated me about this bout of this illness is that people were so mad that I was posting so much about it on Facebook. I didn't even know until two people told me. I was like why aren't they telling me or asking me about it? But no, that's because women like to chat, they like to gossip, they very unfortunately like to find flaws in other people so that they make themselves feel better. I get it, I've fallen into that myself, and thank God I try not to fall into that since my conversion. It is always a temptation. But it was as if these people thought I should stop talking about it so much. That I should stop doing videos, going live or sharing links to hard videos of women out there who experienced this. Well guess what? Two things: 1. It's my Facebook so like me, don't like me, friend me, don't friend me, unfriend me, hide my posts but I am not going to change. And 2. I don't care. Some people write to get through postpartum depression, some people get sucked into it and die, and then there are others like me who TALK about it because it makes me feel better. What they didn't know is that I was doing it all for a reason. I knew that I was going to write this book so I hashtagged the crap out of my postpartum depression posts. When I arose from this jet lag of postpartum depression, I went back to my Facebook and I studied myself from the moment I got it to up until that day. You can all thank (or not thank!) those posts, which basically created the shell for this book. I never would have remembered anything unless I posted as much as I did and unless I hashtagged so yeah, sorry not sorry is how I address that one.

On a more positive note, the amount of great feedback I got was amazing. I got so many people on either my personal Facebook page or my Camaraderie Mom Facebook/Twitter pages. People commending me for speaking so openly about it. People who, like my male tenant, said no one ever talks about this and it is very serious. They were the fuel that ignited my desire to write this book aside from the fact that I would love to have every hospital put something more serious about postpartum depression in their packets to go home with moms. I don't know about you but I have eight packets from eight pregnancies (remember I have a set of twins) and while I have a flood of information about vaccines, cord blood banking, etc. I only have one document on postpartum depression and it is buried at the bottom of the stack of papers. I personally think that if any of these documents need to be front and center it should be the one on postpartum depression, wouldn't you agree?

So in short, while the world may go on not talking about it I hereby declare that I will not shut up about postpartum depression like ever.

CHAPTER 23

Dads Have Postpartum Depression Too

So you know how people say that during pregnancy the fathers can have pregnancy sympathy? They are hungry, they are tired, and who knows, maybe even their stomachs get bigger! Well this may come as a shock to you but men can have postpartum depression too! As WebMD states:

Postpartum depression hits new dads, too. Moreover, male postpartum depression may have more negative effects on some aspects of a child's development than its female counterpart, says James F. Paulson, PhD, of the Center for Pediatric Research at the Eastern Virginia Medical School in Norfolk, Va. Paulson and colleagues reviewed data on more than 5,000 two-parent families with children aged 9 months. They found that one in 10 new dads met standard criteria for moderate to severe postpartum depression.

That's a little shocking, no? But it is true. And think about nowadays, more dads are staying home with the children so it only makes sense. They are sleep deprived! They are run ragged just like moms. So it is only natural that while their hormones may not be out of whack, if they are sleep deprived, which they likely are, then it is like a cesspool for postpartum depression!

My dad told me a personal story about one male who he believed had postpartum depression. He said that he had a sales representative who had not called on his accounts for several weeks and his customers were calling my dad and asking my dad where he was. My dad was unable to reach him by phone so my dad traveled to his territory, went to his home, and found him on a swing rocking his baby and singing lullabies to the baby. The man told my dad that he was having a difficult time working because he felt that he should be at home all the time protecting the baby. After my dad got him some counseling, he was able to return to work. It was the first time that my dad had heard about a male having postpartum depression, which the counselor said it was. Eventually he recovered but he was on a sick leave for a long time and it was all because he had postpartum depression.

So it is very important for us not to forget the dads out there, as they could be struggling with postpartum depression as well!

CHAPTER 24

Yes, We Would Still Have More and More and More

People always ask us if we would have more children and we always have the same answer: we will do whatever God wants. Now that I have had this severe second bout with postpartum depression I feel like they ask the same exact question. We would give the same answer even now.

You have to understand a few things about me. I have always had virtually perfect pregnancies, labors, and deliveries. My old OBGYN practice - which was a team of people and to my knowledge, not devout in any faith though they may be and I just did not know it- they were never surprised when I showed up pregnant so quickly. It became a joke like gee, didn't make it to your yearly visit again huh? And while they knew and I knew that I should go one year without getting pregnant especially after my C-section it just never happened except for after number eight, Joseph. My new doctor who is a devout Catholic also was not surprised by getting pregnant so soon. So you have to understand that none of my doctors ever have told me to stop getting pregnant for any reason.

So some might say, but since this bout of postpartum depression was so severe, don't you think you should take a break and just stop? No. Heck no. Why? For me that is like telling a person who went on a ship and got sea sick they should never go on a ship again. Never enjoy a cruise again? Are you going to let this illness control your life? I'm not. That's like giving in and giving up. However, with that said, I personally could have stopped a long time ago but I don't let my feelings, my wants dictate my life for one sheer fact: I let God dictate my life. If He wants us to have more, we will have more. If He doesn't, we won't. After all, as the saying goes, God only gives us what we can handle, right? I totally disagree with it but anyways...

So yes, as crazy as it sounds we would be open to more children. Whatever happens, happens. We will do our charting best! And who knows, maybe we will get A+s for years or who knows, maybe we will fail miserably. At least if we fail miserably we will get a cute bundle of joy out of it! And if that dark evil postpartum depression creeps back up on us then I will attack it like I have in the past and this time, but no, this sucky illness won't dictate my life like ever.

Conclusion

I hope that this book has helped you or a loved one in some way. My goal was to share my story, which is an ongoing one since I have months or even years left to watch and monitor this illness no matter how normal I feel. I can't predict how long this will last. I can't say that every day will be the same. When you talk to women who share this illness there is one common thread that is shared and that is that it will get better! And that is so true. It will and it does get better. The beginning is hell, sheer hell. The middle is also a type of hell. But then the days get brighter, things seem more manageable and things start to stabilize. Of course you will have your ups and your downs but that is why it is critical to have a good support system. Get help!

I will be honest and say that the days that I was depressed or even just anxious thinking about when the hell would end, I had moments where I was nervous about getting completely better. I imagine that sounds bad but hear me out. When you have lived through something like postpartum depression and when you have a good support system you are somewhat spoiled. For weeks and months having people or even just my husband take care of me is unlike the previous ten plus years of my life. When I get better, will anyone care? Will anyone help? I hate to say it but it is true. I see it in particular with my own family. My family immediately went to all measures to help me in the beginning but now that I am just ok I barely hear from some of them anymore. Do they not realize that I still need help? Do they realize that the reason I got into this mess is because I was doing too much? So what happens when I am completely better and over-doing it again? Will my husband still want to take the baby at night? Will my family still offer to help or will I be left alone like I was before that? It sounds gloomy and I don't mean it to be but that is why having a support system that you can be open with is so important for your entire journey through postpartum depression.

I feel blessed. I feel lucky. This bout of severe postpartum depression may have only lasted less than five months but I can assure you I still have my bad days. I still get depressed. The triggers have changed but I can spot them now because I am more in tune to my body and my surroundings than ever. For that I am grateful to this illness. I know when I can speed up and I know when I should slow down. I know when I am over-stimulated for whatever reason and need to go to a quiet place so I don't lose my cool or "relapse". Yes, in one way I feel like someone who is recovering from something that I didn't ask for but was placed in my lap so to speak. I have people I can talk to, people who can relate and understand me. I have the postpartum progress forum which I am on a lot whether it is for me or to give light to others. I feel the knowledge and the power that has come from this illness and I am ready to pass it on. If no one is there for you, I am. Trust me when I say you can connect with me on Facebook, Twitter, my web page and on the forums. Even if you don't see me I will see you (there).

If you or someone you know suffers from this please reach out for help. Contact your OBGYN, your family doctor, and anyone who can be a support system to you. Don't worry about what it will take to get you better. Just focus on getting better. You may break your own rules like I did, such as taking medication, but if that brings you back to you, to your normal, then that is ok. Remember to rest as much as possible, sleep when you can, and for the love of God, try to take it easy whenever you can! Laundry can wait, house cleaning can wait, and in actuality most things can wait! Enjoy that baby as much as you can and if you can't, just focus on getting better! Trust me, as a Mom of nine children, if you miss a few weeks of their life to take care of you they will be fine and in the long run they, you and your family will be better! Get the help you need, no matter the size little or small, and just remember you are not alone. Somewhere someone else is battling the same thing that you are. They are with you in it! And once you get better, maybe you too can break the stigma around postpartum depression and put a voice to this illness.

Addendum: Poems, Songs, and My Blogs on Postpartum Depression

I found this poem one night when I had been at the tail end of my postpartum depression. I found it because I had recalled reciting a part of it when I was a young girl. To be honest I never read more than the first paragraph because the book I was to practice it from did not have more than that. At any rate, when I read the whole poem as an adult and two time postpartum depression survivor I was floored. It hit home for me and I honestly felt that it should be shared with family members and friends of those who have postpartum depression. Some women want to hide behind the mask of this illness. If people do not see that very mask and try to help then some women do hide when what they really need is help.

Please Hear What I'm Not Saying by Charles C. Finn

Don't be fooled by me.
Don't be fooled by the face I wear
for I wear a mask, a thousand masks,
masks that I'm afraid to take off,
and none of them is me.
Pretending is an art that's second nature with me,
but don't be fooled,
for God's sake don't be fooled.
I give you the impression that I'm secure,

that all is sunny and unruffled with me, within as well as without,
that confidence is my name and coolness my game,
that the water's calm and I'm in command
and that I need no one,
but don't believe me.
My surface may seem smooth but my surface is my mask,
ever-varying and ever-concealing.
Beneath lies no complacence.
Beneath lies confusion, and fear, and aloneness.
But I hide this. I don't want anybody to know it.
I panic at the thought of my weakness exposed.
That's why I frantically create a mask to hide behind,
a nonchalant sophisticated facade,
to help me pretend,
to shield me from the glance that knows.
But such a glance is precisely my salvation, my only hope,
and I know it.
That is, if it's followed by acceptance,
if it's followed by love.
It's the only thing that can liberate me from myself,
from my own self-built prison walls,
from the barriers I so painstakingly erect.
It's the only thing that will assure me
of what I can't assure myself,
that I'm really worth something.
But I don't tell you this. I don't dare to, I'm afraid to.
I'm afraid your glance will not be followed by acceptance,
will not be followed by love.
I'm afraid you'll think less of me,

that you'll laugh, and your laugh would kill me.
I'm afraid that deep-down I'm nothing
and that you will see this and reject me.
So I play my game, my desperate pretending game,
with a facade of assurance without
and a trembling child within.
So begins the glittering but empty parade of masks,
and my life becomes a front.
I idly chatter to you in the suave tones of surface talk.
I tell you everything that's really nothing,
and nothing of what's everything,
of what's crying within me.
So when I'm going through my routine
do not be fooled by what I'm saying.
Please listen carefully and try to hear what I'm not saying,
what I'd like to be able to say,
what for survival I need to say,
but what I can't say.
I don't like hiding.
I don't like playing superficial phony games.
I want to stop playing them.
I want to be genuine and spontaneous and me
but you've got to help me.
You've got to hold out your hand
even when that's the last thing I seem to want.
Only you can wipe away from my eyes
the blank stare of the breathing dead.
Only you can call me into aliveness.
Each time you're kind, and gentle, and encouraging,
each time you try to understand because you really care,

my heart begins to grow wings–
very small wings,
very feeble wings,
but wings!
With your power to touch me into feeling
you can breathe life into me.
I want you to know that.
I want you to know how important you are to me,
how you can be a creator–an honest-to-God creator–
of the person that is me
if you choose to.
You alone can break down the wall behind which I tremble,
you alone can remove my mask,
you alone can release me from my shadow-world of panic,
from my lonely prison,
if you choose to.
Please choose to.
Do not pass me by.
It will not be easy for you.
A long conviction of worthlessness builds strong walls.
The nearer you approach to me the blinder I may strike back.
It's irrational, but despite what the books say about man
often I am irrational.
I fight against the very thing I cry out for.
But I am told that love is stronger than strong walls
and in this lies my hope.
Please try to beat down those walls

with firm hands but with gentle hands
for a child is very sensitive.
Who am I, you may wonder?
I am someone you know very well.
For I am every man you meet
and I am every woman you meet.

The Songs That Saved Me

Since the first few days of my diagnosed postpartum depression was a blur I do not remember which day it was but my girlfriend texted me a song that just put everything into perspective with me. She sent me a link to the YouTube video and the video had a picture of a cross and then the words scrolled by. This was so key for me in those first few days because I could not focus, I could not concentrate. So as I listened to the song I read the words and I could not stop crying. I still can't. I have watched that same video almost every single day since this wave started and all I can do is cry because it speaks to my soul. If you are also riding the postpartum wave with me maybe you too will find comfort in her words:

"Trust In You" by Lauren Daigle

Letting go of every single dream
I lay each one down at Your feet
Every moment of my wandering
Never changes what You see

I've tried to win this war I confess
My hands are weary I need Your rest
Mighty Warrior, King of the fight
No matter what I face, You're by my side

When You don't move the mountains I'm
needing You to move
When You don't part the waters I wish I could
walk through
When You don't give the answers as I cry out to You
I will trust, I will trust, I will trust in You!

Truth is, You know what tomorrow brings
There's not a day ahead You have not seen
So, in all things be my life and breath
I want what You want Lord and nothing less

When You don't move the mountains I'm
needing You to move
When You don't part the waters I wish
I could walk through
When You don't give the answers as I cry out to You
I will trust, I will trust, I will trust in You!

You are my strength and comfort
You are my steady hand
You are my firm foundation; the rock on which I
stand

Your ways are always higher
Your plans are always good
There's not a place where I'll go,
You've not already stood

When You don't move the mountains I'm
needing You to move
When You don't part the waters I wish I
could walk through
When You don't give the answers as I cry out to You
I will trust, I will trust, I will trust in You!

I will trust in You!
I will trust in You!
I will trust in You!

One day while driving the kids to school my oldest son Peter put on this song, which also gave me a great sense of peace while coping with the symptoms of postpartum depression:

"Call on Jesus" by Nicole C. Mullen

I'm so very ordinary
Nothing special on my own
I have never walked on water
I have never calmed a storm
Sometimes I'm hiding away
From the madness around me
Like a child who's afraid of the dark

[Chorus:]
But when I call on Jesus
All things are possible
I can mount on wings like eagles and soar
When I call on Jesus
Mountains are gonna fall

'Cause He'll move heaven
And earth to come rescue me when I call

Lalalala...

Weary brother
Broken daughter
Widowed, widowed lover
You're not alone
If you're tired and
Scared of the madness around you
If you can't find the strength to carry on

[Chorus]

Call Him in the mornin'
In the afternoon time
Late in the evenin'
He'll be there
When your heart is broken
And you feel discouraged
You can just remember that He said
He'll be there

[Chorus x2]

Lalalala...

    Another song that helped me after months of dealing with postpartum depression was one referred to me by my friend, Katie:

"Motion Of Mercy" by Francesca Battistelli

I was poor I was weak
I was the definition of the spiritually
Bankrupt condition
So in need of help

I was unsatisfied
Hungry and thirsty
When You rushed to my side
So unworthy
Still You gave yourself away...

[Chorus]
That's the motion of mercy
Changing the way and the why we are
That's the motion of mercy
Moving my heart

Now I'm filled by a love
That calls me to action
I was empty before now I'm drawn to compassion
And to give myself away

[Chorus]
That's the motion of mercy
Changing the way and the why we are
That's the motion of mercy
Moving my heart

Living for the lost
Loving 'til it hurts
No matter what the cost

Like You loved me first
That's the motion of mercy

God give me strength to give something for nothing
I wanna be a glimpse of the Kingdom that's coming soon

[Chorus]
That's the motion of mercy
Changing the way and the why we are
That's the motion of mercy
Moving my heart

Living for the lost
Loving 'til it hurts
No matter what the cost
Like You loved me first
That's the motion of mercy
Moving my heart
To give yourself away
To give it all away
That's the motion of mercy

    This song came to me later during my wave but the timing of it was perfect:

"Overcomer" by Mandesa

Staring at a stop sign
Watching people drive by
T Mac on the radio
Got so much on your mind
Nothing's really going right

Looking for a ray of hope

Whatever it is you may be going through
I know He's not gonna let it get the best of you

[Chorus:]
You're an overcomer
Stay in the fight 'til the final round
You're not going under
'Cause God is holding you right now
You might be down for a moment
Feeling like it's hopeless
That's when He reminds You
That you're an overcomer
You're an overcomer

Everybody's been down
Hit the bottom, hit the ground
Ooh, you're not alone
Just take a breath, don't forget
Hang on to His promises
He wants You to know

[Chorus]

The same Man, the Great I am
The one who overcame death
He's living inside of You
So just hold tight, fix your eyes
On the one who holds your life
There's nothing He can't do
He's telling you

(Take a breath, don't forget
Hang on to His promises)

[Chorus]

You're an overcomer
You're an overcomer
You're an overcomer

So don't quit, don't give in, you're an overcomer
Don't quit, don't give in, you're an overcomer
Don't quit, don't give in, you're an overcomer
You're an overcomer

    I must say that I have loved Meghan Trainor's music since her first song came out. I had been singing this song for weeks and then one day I realized how much it reminded me of how I felt during the first wave of this illness. For me it was God and His love saving me since only He knew truly how I felt both internally and externally.

"Kindly Calm Me Down" by Meghan Trainor

So cold, alone
Could you be my blanket?
Surround my bones
When my heart feels naked
No strength, too weak
I could use some saving
And you're love's so strong

Like a pill I take it, I take it, I take it

Like a pill, your love, I take it
I take it, I take it
Like a pill, your love, I take it

When my world gets loud, could you make it quiet down?
When my head, it pounds, could you turn down all the sound?
If I lay in pain, by my side would you stay?
If I need you now, would you kindly calm me down?
Oh-oh-oh, oh-oh-oh, would you kindly calm me down?
Oh-oh-oh, oh-oh-oh, would you kindly calm me down?

When my heart's not pure
Would you kill my disease?
And when there's no cure
You are just what I need
When I lose my mind
Would you still remind me?
When I'm feeling lost
Would you come and find me?

I'd take it, I would take it
Like a pill, your love, I take it
I take it, I take it
Like a pill, your love, I take it

When my world gets loud, could you make it quiet down?
When my head, it pounds, could you turn down all the sound?

If I lay in pain, by my side would you stay?
If I need you now, would you kindly calm me down?
Oh-oh-oh, oh-oh-oh, would you kindly calm me down?
Oh-oh-oh, oh-oh-oh, would you kindly calm me down?

When my world gets loud, could you make it quiet down?
When my head, it pounds, could you turn down all the sound?
If I lay in pain, by my side would you stay?
If I need you now, would you kindly calm me down?

When my world gets loud, could you make it quiet down?
When my head, it pounds, could you turn down all the sound?
If I lay in pain, by my side would you stay?
If I need you now, would you kindly calm me down?
Oh-oh-oh, oh-oh-oh, would you kindly calm me down?
Oh-oh-oh, oh-oh-oh, would you kindly calm me down?

My Blogs on Postpartum Depression

I have two blogs that I hold deep to my heart. First is my Camaraderie Mom blog and the second is my religious blog. I have decided to include the blogs that I wrote on postpartum depression here in this chapter. If you would like to follow my blogs you can here:

Camaraderie Mom:
http://camaraderiemom.com/
One Religious Rebel:
https://onereligiousrebel.wordpress.com/

Taming The Postpartum Beast Within You.

I dedicate this post to Bernadette, my beloved friend who is riding my wave of postpartum depression. Thanks for being there, always being a light, and always putting things into spiritual perspective.

I was raised in a different time. A time where kids were allowed to run free outside at any hour without any worry. In one way that is good. In other ways it is not good in that, for people like me, a "wild horse," it is like being set free without a bridle. Some people need "leashes." Some people need "bridles." I am one of those.

In that regard it is no shock to me that -especially with postpartum depression- I have to endure an internal battlefield that may be unlike others. People who are used to having boundaries (because today's environment calls for it) may not have to deal with the type of crazy that people who have been set free and run wild have to endure. It may be my imagination but anyways...

I am so thankful that at a young age I converted and was introduced to people who not only called out the wild horse in need of taming but actually tried to help tame her (me). It is one thing to tame someone from the outside: change the way they look, dress, walk, etc. OK, no biggie. But try changing the inside? Yeah, good luck with that one. And yet, they had success. These holy priests broke through and to be honest I am not nearly as wild as I was or could have been thanks to them. I know, shocking indeed.

With their training, per se, I now know how to try to attempt to tame the postpartum depression beast within me (and trust me it is a beast). One moment super happy; the next moment super mad. One day up; the next day down. One moment enlightened and the next moment I've got nuttin'. However, with prayer and practice one can tame that beast and rein her back in. Prayer, temperance, quiet, meditation, and so many key spiritual practices can kick that beast in the big fat arse!

So here's to all my fellow "wild horses," and to all my fellow people who deal with internal battlefields. May your battle be quick and your victory be perpetual!

Sincerely yours,
One Religious Rebel

What Is Normal?

This sucks. This being postpartum depression. One day up, the next day down. You never know what each day will bring. As the days pass you wonder when you will be back to normal. But as the days pass you almost forget what normal, your normal, is. It's like the pit of postpartum depression was so deep that you forget what it felt like to be normal because well, being normal doesn't take any work and we likely take it for granted.

There will be days that I think I am totally fine and then my daughter will come up to me, wave her hand in front of me, and tell me she is breaking my stare. I was staring? OMG I was, thanks. Something so small as that that I didn't even notice. A blank stare into the nothingness of postpartum depression.

Then there will be other days where I sense it coming on out of nowhere: utter anxiety. The kicker is I have anxiety about absolutely nothing, which makes no sense. But this illness is illogical so what can you do?

I think what I miss most of all about my being normal is that I didn't have to think about being happy or joyful; I just was. I always was well when I wasn't screaming at my kids because they drew on the walls or whatnot! It is mind boggling to me that one has to make an effort to be happy or joyful. One has to do something to cause that feeling in them but I never really had to.

I am not sure if and when my normal will return. I am not sure I will even recognize it. But if it does come and I do remember it to be my normal I will embrace it in the most extraordinary way.

God bless,
JoAnne

Just Keep Swimming (Through postpartum Depression)

I dedicate this to all of my ships, my life jackets. Thank you for helping me and taking care of my family and me!

As I sit here from my hotel room I see the ocean view.

We weren't supposed to get this room. We complained for the wait and now that I am here and we have the view I know it is providential that we got the view.

I sit here with a glass of wine, without any one of my nine children or my husband while he works downstairs. The silence is almost deafening. I sit here, I look out to the ocean, and all I think of is how it reminds me of my postpartum depression.

I look out, forward (not backward) and I see nothing. I see no shore. I see no end in sight. I am sad. Will this end? The anxious feelings I get when I am in public, the mind racing, the irrational thinking. Right now-during the very bad moments-I see no shore!

From my view I look at the waves crashing on the sand. I see some high tides. I see some low tides... I feel like that. Some days are good. Some days are bad. Some days are iffy. All days I ride the wave. Sometimes I go under but I always come up. I have to. I am wired that way. I may come up and be doing a crappy job but thank God I always come up.

I wonder what the point of low tide and high tide is anyways. What was God thinking with that? And yet in the low and high tides of postpartum depression I see, from a religious (and even other) aspect, why we have them. Low tide is a relief. It gives up hope. High tide is painful, a sacrifice but one that reminds us (or me anyways) to slow the hell down.

As I watch the seagulls like they are gonna drown, out of nowhere there is a ship! There is hope. I feel like one of those guys out there, in the deepest darkest hours of my life thank God I saw the ship. Thank God the ship saw me! Thank God the ship re-routed and found me, took care of me. Thank God they tossed me a life jacket, pulled me onto their boat, and took me to shore.

We may not see the end in sight. We may not see the shore but this is one fact for sure: there is ALWAYS a shore. It may be friggin' far and the route may be tough but hell, it is there. So if you are like me do as Dory says and "just keep swimming" through postpartum depression. Seek help and it will find you and then all of your riding the wave and treading water will not be in vain. Who knows? You may save someone else in the process.

God bless,
JoAnne

Moms, be happy to be alive today. Happy Mother's Day!

Moms; be happy to be alive today.

Happy Mother's Day to all the moms out there. I hate to put a crazy title to this but I am living in a crazy world right now. A world where one day is normal and the next is not. I am living in a world of postpartum depression. I am not depressed. But I have the other symptoms. I am off. I have anxiety. My mind races. I can't cope like I used to. Oh my.

You think for having nine kids in 10 years I would have it down pat. I do not. I have never experienced PPD like now. I am grateful for my sane moments. I am grateful when I can play with my kids. I am grateful when I can drive. I am grateful for every

EFFIN thing. Because when you go from totally normal to totally insane you become grateful. Be happy to be alive and normal, moms.

I am happy to be alive today. My baby was born the end of March. After a week of birth I did not think I would live. I felt like I died. In ER terms I did not but to me I was so close to death.

Here I am and I am coping with this. And all I want to say is that for those of you who are normal out there, you Moms, please embrace this; your motherhood. For those of you struggling like me right now, there is not a lot to be said. But I salute you. Keep going. You've got this. It will end!

To all mothers, no matter what, the times when you feel overdone, overworked, underpaid, remember your reward is in heaven. I believe it is. You are not doing this for nothing. Despite what the world says, you are forming people AND THAT IS THE MOST EFFIN IMPORTANT JOB IN THE WORLD.

#nuffsaid #shortestblogever #happymothersday

God bless,
JoAnne

Listen to your body, Momma...

I had postpartum depression with my fourth child. Had I listened to my body I would have caught it sooner, not at 3.5 months postpartum. Had I listened to my body I would not have postpartum now with the delivery of my ninth child who was born six weeks ago.

Nurses and medical staff always say, "Listen to your body." Well damn, they are right on. I am an idiot. I should have listened to brother arse as I call her. I didn't but I am here to talk about it nonetheless.

Reference my last blog in order to know what you are dealing with here. I explained part one of the journey I have had with postpartum depression so here is round two or shot two (it feels like a shot!).

I am NOT a medical professional even if I want to be. I am a mom. I am a wife. I am a patient. And I am experiencing ups and downs like you can't imagine. Maybe you can benefit from my (continuing) story.

If I would have listened to my body I never would have stressed out or reacted about the fact that two days postpartum I was going to lose the house of our dreams.

If I would have listened to my body I would have said to myself, "screw it, who cares?" and enjoyed my baby. I did not because I am a masochist. I did not because while I was in the hospital having the time of my life my home was in disarray because of the potential move.

I got home and I did not do a thing physically but I stressed mentally and emotionally. I cried a lot. A whole friggin' lot. I could not sleep. All I could think of was how I promised my eight kids this house and how I had to get it. How would I undo my old house if we had to stay there? So much was packed. Insanity.

But I did it. I got through. We got the house. The day before we closed we spent the whole day loading U-Hauls. The next day we emptied the entire home into a new home. It was a happy disaster. I drank. A LOT. That is how I cope. Choose your fix: anxiety meds or alcohol. I chose boxed Chardonnay and yes, it must be BOXED.

The next day I get up very early after little sleep and starting working. And then, in my twisted mind I think I must go to Mass. Mass? Yes, Mass. Um, I could have been excused. I take my son to Mass and upon entering the church the stimulation is too much for me. It hits me. Like lightning bolts. I smile at my son and get him to his gig and I remove myself from the main church into the foyer. I kiss the cross on my keychain, crumble to the floor literally, and cry. I know what has happened. I have postpartum depression and now there is no turning back.

I go to the car to sleep. I can't sleep. I wait for my son thinking I really shouldn't drive home. I should have listened to my body, which was blaring at me for so long: STOP. EFFING STOP. No friggin' lying; it said the F bomb and I don't curse. My body cursed.

I get home and eventually end up in the ER. And here I am 6 weeks later VERY HAPPY that I am alive to tell this story. Listen to your body, Momma.

If I would have listened to my body it would have said:

Stop.
Sleep.
Sleep more.
Nap.
Nap more.
Ask for help.
Stop doing so much.
Take your multi vitamin.
Take your b-complex INTRAVENOUSLY.
Take your thyroid pill (which your doc cut off). Take a walk.
Exercise.
Get sunlight.
Listen to music.
Cut out (TOO MUCH) alcohol.
Cut out coffee.
Cut out caffeine.
Cut out chocolate.
Cut out anything with ANY amount of caffeine like tea
Call your doctor.
Call your OTHER doctor.
Call your nurse.
Call your sitter.

Call ANYONE who can help.
Talk. Talk to anyone who will listen.
Remember that those thoughts, the crazy ones, are IRRATIONAL. Do not act on them.
Don't think you're a doc and cut or increase your meds. You are a mere human. Stick to their rules.
Get you time. Whatever that is. Facial, massage, pedi, date night. Do it. Credit is there for a reason; buy now, pay later.
Research and share. Learn what's going on and share if it makes you feel better.

There is so so so much more I could have listened to in my body. Now I am tuned in to it and I am never ever letting go. Your body tells you what you need. I believe it with all my heart. Had I caught it sooner I think I could have saved myself and others a lot of trouble. It is what it is. I take the good from the bad and I move forward. I am blessed. I am alive. And this is my story, which will be vividly monitored for a year since this postpartum depression can last a year from the baby's birth date.

God bless,
JoAnne

The day it all came crashing down...

It felt like a gust of wind that came from out of nowhere; it suffocated me and brought me to the ground, crumbled on the church floor.

Think. Pray. How do I get my son and myself home? I need sleep.

Go to the car. There's no noise in the car. The Church has too much stimulation. OK.

I will just take a nap in the car until Mass is over and my son is finished with altar serving. Set alarm, only I can't sleep.

Should I drive home? Don't overreact.

I will drive home and just tell my son to keep me distracted. It is four miles only four miles away. You can do this.

Finally, at home. Honey, I must sleep. I am going to bed.

Bed, great. But no, my mind races. Alleluia is played in my mind thousands of times and I can't shut it off.

Honey, I can't sleep. Bring me my pump. I pump because I have to keep up my supply.
What is wrong with me as I sit on the floor of my new home that has no furniture? Did I eat today? I

do not know. Why don't I know? OMG did I eat today? No, no I didn't.

Honey, I need food; bring me crackers. I eat one cracker as if it were fifty. I crumble to the floor desperate to know what is wrong with me. Wait, you had this. This is postpartum depression. F%^&!

Something else is wrong with me. Honey, come here. Honey call 911.

You don't need an ambulance JoAnne; you are having a panic attack.

No, I need an ambulance. Maybe it's my thyroid. I am not taking my pills because they stopped them after birth. Maybe it's my blood pressure? Too high? Too low? Just call, damn it.

I will give you a Xanax.

A Xanax? Says me who never takes any drugs. YES, YES, give me a Xanax.

Five minutes later... why isn't it working? It takes 20 minutes. OK, call 911, something is seriously wrong with me.

Is he on the phone with 911 or is he faking it and talking with his Mom? Is that the police or your mom? You better have called 911.

Yes, I did.

Well, why the hell is it so slow?

Police show up, I have gotten changed, got my pump, got my wallet and my purse, and I am ready to go.

Ma'am, you were not in cardiac arrest so the ambulance will be here soon but not blaring.

Are you kidding me? Well I could have been dead and I could be dead in a minute because you're not in my body dude.

Thirty minutes later ambulance arrives. Can you walk out? I was ready to walk out a long time ago.

Bye, honey, call sitter. Don't argue; call sitter. Meet me at the hospital; I need you there.

I enter the ambulance and the guy wants to talk to me. Xanax kicks in and the edge is off. Thank God! Vitals checked and I am ok. OK, I think I am going to live.

At this point I want to sleep and all he wants to do is talk to me about my fascinating life. I am too nice to shut him down, so we chat.

We arrive at the hospital and I immediately tell the nurse I know my problem: I am a mom of nine kids ages 9 and under, I had a baby on 3.21 and on 4.1 I moved into a new house and took everything from the last home with me. My house is in disarray,

I am sleep-deprived, dehydrated, and I have severe postpartum depression. Ideally I would like you to give me fluids and knock me out. The nurse then agrees with my diagnosis but waits for the doctor.

While she waits she too wants to talk about my life. I entertained her because Xanax is great and I feel safe in the hospital. She tells me we are blessed because she can't get pregnant. I launch into Felix-fix-it from Wreck-it-Ralph and immediately tell her about my doctor, Dr. Kyle Beiter and the Gianna Center. I give her all the info, which she takes down. I tell her I know two people for sure who could not get pregnant until they went to him. She says who is the patient, you or me? as she smiles gratefully.

The doctor comes in and agrees with my diagnosis then launches into our lives and he jokes with 'da hubby and tells him he looks like John Mayer. Are we really having this conversion? OK. He said since the Xanax worked I will give you a script and you should go to your OBGYN or follow up with him. And, hey, get some fluids and rest. Gee thanks. Why am I here then? I think in my head.

I arrive home to a bunch of people. It was a little overwhelming. I just wanted to go to bed. Then my friend talks about her postpartum psychosis and I get freaked out in my head. Bad timing to talk about it.

They leave and I go to bed, but sure enough, I can't sleep. I call my OBGYN. He asks me about my thoughts and I tell him all that is going on in my mind and body. He suggests progesterone. YES, GOD, YES! I have heard of that. Shoot. I am so stupid for not taking it right away after giving birth, like my friend told me to.

Husband arrives at new pharmacy and pharmacy is closed. Great. Thanks, Lord. Doesn't open until 8 or 9 the next day. That felt like an eternity.

That first night is a blur, but I remember freaking out, and I think I took another Xanax. That was the scariest day of my life.

Fast forward. It has been fourteen days since then and in that time period, I feel as if I have experienced every one of the senses so intensely. Sights, sounds, touch, tastes, smells... Seeing things that aren't there. Seeing people's mouths move like you can lip-read. Hearing things that are insane. Hearing things magnified in stereo. Wanting to touch and yet not wanting to be touched. Things not tasting the same or right or good for you or having no taste for anything at all. Smelling intently every smell or not smelling anything.

Thoughts. Having every single crazy insane thought I could ever have and yet knowing it is totally irrational thinking.

Anxiety and fear about everything. ABSOLUTELY everything! Holding the baby, bathing the baby, driving again, doing normal activities again, and being alone. Every fear out there I have had.

Every day has gotten better, and I now know what triggers set me off. I am trying to take things one day at a time, one job or task at a time. I know what I need to do to get better; after all I have been through this before. I had this with Bella, but Bella was mild. Like in DEF con levels, if 5 is the worst, Bella was a 1 and this one is a 6 knowing that 6 is greater than 5.

I will get better. I must get better. My husband needs a wife. My children need their mother. And now, I have a new desire, one I have had before but not as intently: I need to get the word out on postpartum depression. If no one else will speak out about it, I will. It's too important not to talk about. So yes, this illness won't silence me because it needs a voice and I am going to be its voice screaming from the rooftops.

-The victim, but not for long...

The Dark Night of The Soul

I am floored. I simply cannot believe I have not blogged on here since February. It makes me downright sad. However, I must forgive myself because the last few weeks and month have been a blur.

I have experienced the dark night of the soul many times over. I remember it vividly when I was younger and I remember thinking it was my penance, my purification for all of my past sins. I still hated going through it but I remember thinking there would be a reward to the suffering.

If you have not read Saint John of the Cross and his take on the dark night of the soul, I encourage you to read it. He nails it. He is one of my favorite saints.

I remember at the beginning of my conversion a great friend telling me to always remember that time because later in life there would be a dark night. She was right. There have been many dark nights and I do remember what it felt like to first fall in love with God, to discover Him and to feel His presence like never before. That time, and that very memory has saved me through many a trial.

We live in a world that does not like to suffer. People do not understand suffering. People understand quick fixes. People do not see the benefit of suffering. However, Christ is the perfect example of why one should suffer. In His suffering there is redemption. In His suffering there is forgiveness of sins, and oh yeah, forgiveness of sins OF THE ENTIRE WORLD. So there is a benefit to suffering even if we do not see it or feel it.

I will be honest and say that I have never ever experienced the dark night of the soul like I did this past month. It was hell on earth. I thought I would die. I thought I would go to hell. I knew there was a God but I could only see evil, darkness, and death. I prayed and yet I prayed not with words. I prayed with my soul. Sometimes we have no words. Sometimes we are desperate. I was desperate. I communicated with God without words. I communicated with pain. I communicated with darkness. And He, for whatever reason, pulled me through it and into the light.

When you experience that type of darkness it is true that the light seems ever brighter. It as if you are a child just opening your eyes for the first time. You are in awe of your surroundings. You are grateful for the light. You embrace it like never before.

It is in that way that I am actually grateful for the dark night of the soul. It puts everything into perspective. We take life for granted. We take things for granted. But when you are in the darkness you can't see anything. Yet, when you return to that light everything is anew.

I do not know why God shows me His mercy and His love in this way but I will take it. I will run with it. I will embrace it, and if ever a dark night comes again, though I may be afraid, I trust in Him and I will say bring it on, baby.

Sincerely yours,
One Religious Rebel

References

Mayo Clinic:
http://www.mayoclinic.org/diseases-conditions/postpartum-depression/basics/symptoms/con-20029130

Merriam-Webster:
http://www.merriam-webster.com/dictionary/depression

WebMD:
http://www.webmd.com/depression/postpartum-depression/news/20080506/men-also-get-postpartum-depression

Postpartum Progress:
http://www.postpartumprogress.com/

www.ingramcontent.com/pod-product-compliance
Lightning Source LLC
LaVergne TN
LVHW051842080426
835512LV00018B/3020